Lyme Disease Sucks

the trauma, the truth & the triumph

Leonie Shanahan

Disclaimer

The author is not a doctor or health practitioner. This book is not medical advice. All information contained within is of the nature of general comment only, based on the author's experience, and is not in any way recommended as individual advice. This book is provided for informational and educational purposes. Many of the treatments presented are experimental and not medical approved. This book is not intended as a substitute for professional medical advice, treatment, diagnosis or cure of any specific kind of medical condition. The reader should consult a medical practitioner/qualified health professional in matters relating to his/her health, and particularly with respect to any symptoms that may require diagnosis or medical attention. Should any reader choose to make use of the information contained herein, this is their decision, and authors and publishers do not assume any responsibility whatsoever under any condition or circumstance. It is recommended that the reader obtain their own medical advice.

Published with Support by Author Express 2021

www.edibleschoolgardens.com.au

A catalogue record for this book is available from the National Library of Australia.

ISBN:
978-1-925471-54-0 (pbk)
978-1-925471-55-7 (ebk)

Editor: Caryn Stevens
Book cover design and formatting services by SelfPublishinglab.com

Dedication

I dedicate this book to my sister,

Anne-Maree Shanahan.

I would not be alive today without her

never-ending unconditional love,

financial support,

and mental health pep talks.

$1 will be donated to
Lyme Disease Association of Australia
for every copy sold

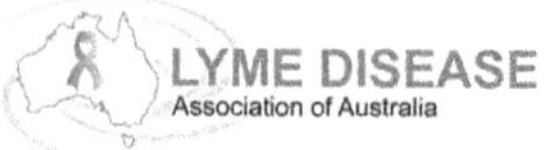

Contents

Foreword

Sharing our story can be both healing for ourselves, and supportive of the healing of others. In *Lyme disease Sucks: the trauma, the truth, & the triumph*, Leonie Shanahan has certainly achieved the latter, and we hope also the former. Leonie courageously shares her journey of illness, struggle and perseverance. She describes the costs that Lyme disease imposed on her life, the options she faced, the choices she made, what helped, and what didn't help. Leonie also acknowledges how much she valued the support and understanding she received from friends and loved ones.

Where do Lyme and associated diseases come from? Ticks. They are blood-feeding parasites that are often found in tall grasses where they wait to attach to a passing host, such as humans or dogs. Ticks can be found in most wooded or forested regions throughout the world and often latch on to shoes or clothes, before working their way up your clothing, until they find a prime piece of exposed skin. There are at least 14 different types of bacteria that cause Lyme disease identified world-wide, and currently research is underway in Australia to isolate exactly the type of tick, and the specific bacteria, that is causing it here. Most of the ticks that infect people with Lyme disease are in the nymph, or immature stage of development, and are about the size of a poppy seed, which means that many people do not remember a tick bite. The BEST prevention against Lyme and associated infections is to: a) prevent tick bites b) check for ticks after being outside c) remove ticks safely d) watch for any rashes, flu-like symptoms or other reactions, and get immediate, informed medical care. Lyme disease websites, such as the Lyme Disease Association of Australia, contain more detailed information.

Unfortunately, an estimated half a million people are suffering from Lyme and associated illnesses in Australia. Many cannot obtain appropriate medical care and suffer intolerable discrimination. They're told it's all in their heads. This situation exists because of legacy thinking, denial, ignorance in research, and the apathy of policy makers to properly investigate the phenomena. The impacts affect real people. These are the 'abandoned ones', and this book is an example of their story. The issues that surround the Lyme disease debate in Australia are complex, but it's crucial that the medical and research communities recognise both the complexity of the issue and the illness and burdens they impose upon individuals, their families, and society. By working together, we can design solutions for what has been described as 'the first epidemic of climate change'.

The journey to recovery through Lyme and associated diseases can be a long and difficult one, and each person's path to healing is unique. It's important to remember that there is no 'one size fits all' treatment protocol This book describes Leonie's experience of being on this journey and helps raise awareness of this debilitating illness. What this story teaches us is to persevere, learn as much as we can, nurture those suffering with these illnesses, and finally, to never give up hope. Thank you, Leonie.

The Lyme Disease Association of Australia.
The LDAA is a small yet powerful registered charity and Australia's peak patient body. We advocate on behalf of patients for accurate information about the illness, well-researched prevention programs and clinical studies, appropriate diagnostic and treatment guidelines, and also provide patient support.

Abundant Gratitude

(Acknowledgements)

My heartfelt gratitude to my core support group that were my anchor from day one, long before I was even officially diagnosed: Karen Cormack, Fiona Ball, Jenny Manson, Anne-Maree Shanahan, and Costa Georgiadis. I could not have survived without you all. My heart swells remembering your constant backing with words, actions, and love.

I also want to send a special thank you to Tansy Grant, who joined the team later in my journey, but is no less appreciated.

To my daughters, Melika and Fedora. I know it's been difficult for you to have a mum with an energy-sucking disease. But despite everything, you've created the most amazing lives for yourselves, and I'm proud of you. I love you both very much.

To the many people who cannot be named, who went well beyond the 'consultation' time to get me through the day. Unfortunately, I'm unable to mention the doctors and natural and alternative medicine practitioners, who want to stay under the radar. But you all know who you are, and I constantly express my absolute gratitude.

I'm forever grateful to the huge number of friends, associates, gardeners, neighbours, healers, and some people I've never met before in my life, who came to my aid.

To all the healers at the Cooroy Lotus Wellbeing Centre who worked on and with me every Monday, and sometimes during the week, too. I needed your safe haven, loving support, healing and regular contact where I could express exactly how I was feeling (usually with tears) and be 'held' by you all. Especially grateful to Jenny, Margaret, Michelle, Roslyn, and Trevor. You've gently taken my hand and helped me discover healing and spirituality, and the knowledge that there's something so much bigger than we are out there, waiting to hold us. We just need to ask.

A special thank you to this wonderful group of awesome people: Mike, Sharon, Mikayla, Jane, Rashmi, Eddie, Sandeep, Charein, Steve, Marcia, Mark Thomas, Amina Eastman, Greg Gralton, Phil McManus, Andy Pike, Skye Duncan, Robin Kerr, David Weir, Tracey Ollett, Jean Sheahan, and Margie Thomson; my friends Brit Ballard, Carole Milroy, Jen L., Tracey Farrow, Sue Rowse, Bevan McLeod, and Jade Woodhouse; my neighbours, Don and Fran; my nieces, Mia, Josie, and Steph, Keryn Rose, who activated my water with healing energy each day; Merryl and Ted, who always had a toolbox of support and remedies for me; the women at HBOT Noosa; Tracey Hatchard, who when I mentioned the idea of writing my story, fuelled me on by not only believing in what I had to offer the world, but also helping to fund it; my Permaculture Noosa friends, who gardened on my organic property when I could not; and Frank Ondrus, for saving me.

To my super-nurturing colonics queen, Beth Beaden, and my health guide, walking encyclopedia, and constant support, Rasunah Alston. Thank you so much.

Much gratitude to those who were praying and meditating for me. You may not think it's much, but for me to know this was happening was so enormously soul lifting.

I want to thank the friends who gave me a roof over my head when I needed one: Tohm Hajncl, Carole Milroy, Colleen Birchel, Penny and Lindsay Foster, Noely and Stephen Neate, and Wendy O'Halloran.

To Lorraine, who let me bounce off wording and sentences, and also had the task of reading the drafts of this book over and over again. I'm incredibly grateful for your 'word wisdom' and enthusiastic support.

To Caryn, my editor, who lives in the U.S.A. I swear you stay up all night to answer my questions. I laughed when one of your first comments was noting the excessive amount of times I'd written *I'm so exhausted!* You're so easy to work with, and you quickly understood where I was coming from. We became a team, ebbing and flowing. Caryn, you are so efficient with language. Thanks for the banter along the way and bringing clarity to my story. (*Now let's see how my editor alters this one. Best editor ever!!)*

I LOVE you all with all of my HEART. I could not have completed this journey without you.

Introduction

I wrote this book for people to understand that Lyme disease is real. It has multiple symptoms that vary daily, which are totally unpredictable. A Lyme sufferer rarely looks sick, which adds to the myth that we are 'fine'. Oh, how untrue that statement is!

This book is my story. I apologise about all the swearing, but in the beginning, I was experiencing such pain, both physical and mental, that I stopped caring about being polite.

To my fellow Lyme patients and friends, I'm here to tell you that you're not alone. I want to give you hope and courage to keep going. It may well be the toughest journey of your life, and certainly not one you would have chosen, but we're in this together, and I hope you come out the other end happy and healthy. I'm living proof that it's possible.

While my journey was hard on so many levels, with symptoms pushing me to the point of wanting to end it all, I acknowledge that there are many more people suffering much worse symptoms every minute of the day. I know of Lyme patients having seizures, who are confined to a wheelchair, who've lost their ability to talk, and are bedridden.

My journey may even look like a walk in the park compared to other people's experiences. The cruellest part for me is not being acknowledged or supported by my government or the Australian medical system. So often, we hit a brick wall of "It's not in this country," and it's assumed we're lying and making it up. We are not. Lyme is being contracted here in large numbers. There's an estimated 10,000 people every year in Australia, and 400,000 in the U.S.A.

Why doesn't our government acknowledge that Lyme disease affects so many people? I believe there may be a couple of reasons, but the main one is that there's no financial incentive for Big Pharma to be involved. Except in cases of acute Lyme, drugs rarely help. Chronic Lyme patients mostly require natural supplements to rebuild and support their body and immune system, plus psychological support...not anti-depressants. Rehabilitation involves multiple healing modalities, which are often not acknowledged as legitimate treatments for a legitimate illness.

I hope in the near future this will change. Maybe a politician or someone within the medical community will read this, gain genuine compassion for Lyme sufferers, and work to establish healthcare and financial assistance.

To become well again, you need commitment, dedication, and courage. You'll have to step outside your comfort zone and find an inner strength you didn't know you had, but please understand that you will be rewarded with having a life again.

As well as taking you through my journey of different treatments, I have included my daily routines, which you may choose to use as a guide. There's also a list of suggestions as to how your friends, family, and support people can help you when you're sick, as often they may avoid you, because they don't know what to do or how to behave. To these people, I say, "We need you more than ever! Even the smallest gestures mean so much."

Have I 'cured' myself of Lyme completely? Definitely not. But I have come further than I ever expected and can again live a good life. I can honestly say I'm the happiest I have ever been ... ever!! Go figure that one out. (Hint: the answers are in the book.)

I will continue seeking out new treatments and following the latest research to build an even stronger body, brain, mind and spirit. I'm addicted to feeling good and living the most amazing life.

And you can be, too.

Healing Hugs
Leonie

CHAPTER 1

The Call

My beautiful white Maltese Shih Tzu, Potcy, waits patiently for me to wake up, so he can go outside for a play. It's 9 February 2015 in Cooroibah, which is a country area near Noosa on Queensland's Sunshine Coast, Australia. It's a hot summer's day, and there's nothing but blue skies.

I grab my large stainless-steel bowl and head out to my organic garden that provides healthy food for three meals a day. When I get there, I collect greens for the guinea pigs and chat to them. "Hello, guineas! Did you have a good sleep?" Then I open the hatch door for my three cute little bantam chooks to come out of their pen and greet them as well. "Good morning, girls. How about you lay some eggs for me today?'" Potcy and I then walk through the undulating rows of organic food, cross the small bridge, and head to the food forest and the freshwater lagoon at the end of my 1.5-acre property.

The water is my solace. It's peaceful and gives me a place for me to cry, scream, and close my eyes while I let the sun fill my soul with hope. After throwing a stick into the water and Potcy retrieving it, a game he could play forever, we get into the canoe and go for a gentle paddle on the water with Potcy the captain of the ship.

Our sailing adventures over, we walk back to the house to make breakfast, when my phone rings. It's the doctor's nurse. She says, "Your results are back from the U.S.A. The doctor wants to see you at 10.30 a.m."

I think my heart has stopped beating. My blood was sent to the U.S.A. for some answers about my ongoing declining health, and for the past two months, I've dreaded receiving this call.

This is it. Whatever those results say, is my destiny. I'm shaking and crying, but there's no one to talk to. I'm home alone. My two daughters, Fedora, who just turned twenty-one, and Melika, sixteen, stayed at their father's last night. So, I text my sister, Anne-Maree, in Victoria. It's more like a telegram in its brief wording:

Test back. Dr appointment at 10.30. Can't stop shaking. Crying.

It's a thirty-minute drive to the doctor's clinic, but for some strange reason, I feel drawn to the volunteer-run healing centre I discovered last week. I leave home early, so I can go there first and join their meditation. I cry silently through the whole thing, and the lady next to me gently takes my hand and holds it in her lap.

I leave and walk the two blocks to the doctor's clinic, where I try to pull myself together by taking some deep breaths. Then I dry my eyes and walk in. I know everyone well, as I've been a regular patient for two years. The receptionist, knowing I keep copies of all my medical results, says to me, "I've done a copy of the results for you." In that moment, the world seems to go in s-l-o-w motion, as this lady with the friendly face hands me a thick report.

I glance down to see that on the front page is the dreaded, feared word: POSITIVE. My world crashes. I know from two months of extensive research that getting a positive on your report is really difficult, and there's one on the first page.

I have Lyme disease.

CHAPTER 2

Facing Reality

I tell the receptionist that I'll wait outside for the doctor. Before I reach the door, the tears are pouring down my face, and the receptionist is right behind me. I sit outside on the garden edge, and she has her arm around my shaking body as I sob and sob and sob and keep saying, "How am I going to look after my daughter? How am I going to do this on my own?"

The nurse comes out to support and comfort me, which allows the receptionist to go back to her desk. I laugh silently as the she makes me a cup of tea. It's so Irish. 'A cuppa fixes everything!'

When I finally see the doctor, I don't really remember anything she says. It's all a blank. I think I have some shell shock going on, but from what I can piece together, I have Lyme disease and multiple Lyme co-infections.

She's so kind and gentle, and spends a lot of time with me. She explains the process and the prescriptions for antibiotics I'll need to take as I vaguely nod in agreement with whatever she says and the printer spits out prescriptions. When the nurse comes in, they both offer support and say they will start a Lyme support group for me.

My appointment over, I walk out to reception, still crying and numb as I pay the bill. I can't stop crying and struggle to put one foot in front of the other. My sister has left numerous worried texts and is waiting for an answer. I send a vague message: *Bad results. Got the lot—Lyme.*

I go back to the healing centre for a massage. When I walk in, they're so concerned. Tears are pouring down my face, I'm shaking and can't speak. Finally, I say, "I've got Lyme disease." Saying it out loud to someone makes it even more real.

I cry through the massage, and then Margaret, a reiki lady and the one who'd held my hand during the mediation, gives me a treatment to calm me down. But it has minimal impact. I cannot face the world. I stay there, not knowing what to do next. I look a mess ... I am a mess. I'm in the kitchen of the centre, when another healer asks me, "Do you need a hug?" Tears stream down my face as I nod *YES.*

My sister is still texting me. It must be hard for her being so far away and knowing I'm falling apart. She tells me to call a friend and get them to meet me, so I text my friend from yoga, Pat, who lives not far away. I tell her I can't face being seen by anyone, because I look a washed-out mess, so we meet at the back of an old museum in Cooroy. It's mid-afternoon by this stage. Pat just listens to me as I express my fears about the future and offers hugs and support.

My niece, Mia, who's flown up from Victoria for Fedora's birthday celebration, has been staying with me. I text her and make up some excuse why she should stay with my girls at their dad's house. Then I text my sister to let her know I'm home and numb, but have stopped crying. There are no tears left. I have a bath and go to bed.

The next day, I lie in bed in the foetal position. The thoughts running through my head on a continuous loop are:

- What am I going to do?
- How am I going to do this?
- How can I be a mother for my girls?
- When Mia arrives, at first I pretend I'm fine, but I know I have to tell her. And when I do, I make it sound light and like there's nothing to worry about. She gives me a big, long hug and asks, "Will you move back home?" We'll look after you." 'Home' is Bendigo Victoria. I tell her how sweet it is for her to offer but that I need to remain where I am.
- When I talk to Melika on the phone, she senses something is wrong, but their dad won't let them return, as he wants them to spend time with his relatives. I ask Mia not to tell them.

When my daughters return the next day, I let them know what's going on and again attempt to downplay it. They don't look worried or upset. They've watched my health decline over the years, but I hide so much from them, as I don't want them to worry. They shouldn't have to carry that.

CHAPTER 3

The Project

Fedora goes back to Brisbane for university, Mia flies home to Bendigo in Victoria, and Melika, who lives with me, goes back to her final year of high school.

For days, the foetal position in bed is my survival mode. The only time I leave it is to care for Melika, the guinea pigs, chooks, and Potcy dog, and then I sit by the water staring at it, hoping for answers.

Why, why, why???

I've been doing good in the world. I have my dream job creating edible school garden programs that teach children how to grow and eat healthy, organic food, I'm creating community gardens at social housing units and mental health facilities, and I'm teaching people how to live better. Why has the universe been so cruel and stopped me?

I love my work. I love helping people, and now I'll have to walk away from it all, because I spend most of my day sleeping and dealing with a long list of other symptoms.

I know that the current program for treating Lyme, multiple antibiotics at once for one or two years, is going to make me real sick. I keep thinking, *How can I do this to Melika, who's going into her final year of school? She wants top marks. How can she possibly study while her mother is throwing up in the toilet from her treatment?* This thought plays round and round in my head, until I decide I can't do this to her. I can't take the antibiotics. I'll have to do it naturally somehow.

While once again curled up in bed, out of the fog of my memory, I remember what the doctor said to me when we first saw the results: "Leonie, your body is so strong! You should be sooooo sick!" And I thought, *I AM sooooo sick*. But I also understand what she meant. On TV, Lyme patients are often shown in wheelchairs and having seizures.

Then comes the realisation: *Oh f***, I don't want that!*

So I say to myself, *Leonie, you're outstanding with projects. It's what you do best. You're great at connecting with people and finding solutions. Make Lyme disease your project. Go out and connect with people in other countries where Lyme is recognised, and find out what they do to get well. Discover natural solutions, and then help other people get healthy.*

With this epiphany, I uncurl and put one foot out of the bed, and then the other (*ouch*!). Then I take my first slow, painful steps to having a purpose and a reason to get well.

My decision to not do antibiotics has given me a breather from people pressuring me to take them. They understand my reason and can't really argue with it. Plus, I now have the space I need to research further and tap into the incredibly experienced doctors and natural medicine doctors/chiropractors, mainly in America, who are providing the latest information. In Australia, Lyme isn't recognised as a disease, and our government doesn't allow doctors to treat it as Lyme. Most wouldn't even know what it is, let alone how to treat it.

The current evidence appears to not support long-term use of antibiotics for chronic Lyme, as it will cause more problems than it solves. An acute patient who's just received a tick bite (or a cat flea, mosquito, midge, sand-fly, or March bite), and has a reaction, needs antibiotics immediately. There's only a small window of opportunity to stop the Lyme and its co-infections before it gets inside your cells and causes havoc. And believe me, you don't want a chronic Lyme disease condition. My doctor would prefer I take the drugs but understands where I'm coming from and is supporting me and waiting.

My mother isn't supportive of my choices. Every time I phone her, the first thing she says is: "Have you started the antibiotics yet?" It doesn't matter how much evidence I give her that drugs won't work for me or share what I'm doing. She refuses to listen. It annoys and upsets me. Mum goes on to say, once again, that her hairdresser knows someone who took antibiotics for Lyme, and it worked! I call that the gospel according to hairdressers (no offence to hairdressers. I do value you).

Thank goodness for Anne-Maree, who's always been there for me. She's five years older and is such a supportive sister. I have needed her so much. In addition to her, I have five other siblings who I email and let them know I'll need their support. None of them live close by, so the best they can do is wish me luck.

Yes. I could sure use some of that right about now.

CHAPTER 4

Origins

My Lyme disease didn't just happen. It's been building momentum. I originally got the tick bite in 1999 while visiting a friend in Wamuran, near Caboolture, Queensland. She lived in the country and had long grass around her home. A couple of days later, I asked a friend we were visiting to check my back near my bra strap, as it was irritating me, and she not so calmly screamed, "*You have a tick! Dogs die from ticks!!*" My first thought was, *I'm not a dog, so I shouldn't die!*" But really, that was the entirety of my knowledge about them.

She then sprayed my back with insect repellent and raced me to the doctor, who was quite amused by the size of the tick. He then invited his colleagues to come in and check it out, as apparently it was quite fat from being "well fed." After he removed it, the doctor said I might experience some reactions but gave me no further information. You'd think I would have felt the tick earlier, but as an exhausted mother, many things just slip past you. And please note: do NOT ever spray a tick on your body with insect repellent, as this will cause it to react and expel more toxins into you.

At the time, my husband and I were doing a caravan trip with our two young children, and we continued travelling north. My back did swell up for nearly a month, but otherwise I just felt the usual exhaustion of motherhood. The habit of needing an afternoon sleep probably increased over the next ten years, and when I'd occasionally say to my doctor, "I get so tired," he would say I was a busy person doing the school garden program, giving talks, and running kids around, so that probably explained it.

In 2011, I made the decision to leave my husband. And although I'd been relieved that I was finally taking action, I was a nervous wreck. First, I had to tell the kids, knowing it would shatter their world. And second, I hadn't been on my own for twenty-seven years, and since having children, I'd let go of keeping a handle on our finances, internet suppliers, and other skills that were required for running a household.

I purchased a 1.5-acre property with two dwellings that I could develop into a permaculture property and pushed myself harder. Plus, now I had a magnificent permaculture dream to evolve as well.

In May 2014, after a busy weekend working a couple of events, plus organising and then dismantling a huge number of plants and displays, I had my first meltdown at the doctor's office. She just told me to take antidepressants. I didn't agree with her, and she didn't take too kindly to my thoughts. Without another option, I continued as I was, going to naturopaths, but eventually it all came crashing down.

In July of that same year, I was at the Queensland Garden Expo, the major garden event in Australia and my biggest event each calendar year. I was on the horticultural advice stand when a fellow horticulture person started pushing me about my life, not in a friendly way, but in a gossiping manner. I told her quite firmly that I didn't want to speak about it. Apparently, that fuelled the fire for further interrogation, and the harassment continued. That's when

I cracked. I got up and ran. Another colleague who'd witnessed my distress, stopped me and gave me a hug. When she asked me what was wrong, I gave a vague answer and took off again, hoping and praying I wouldn't bump into anyone else.

I was aiming for the sanctuary of the car park, which I knew would be deserted this time of day, and hid in the corner where I cried for hours. Sometime later, I managed to pull myself together to present a gardening workshop, which was thankfully outside, so I could leave my sunglasses on. I have no memory of what I said, but people applauded at the end, so I guess I did all right.

Afterward, I drove home in a state. Potcy greeted me warmly, which reminded me that I'd organised the neighbours to mind him overnight, as I was going to a horticulture function that evening.

I didn't want the neighbours seeing me all torn up, so I had to pull myself together somehow, drop the dog to them, and get to the function. This required me drawing on every resource in my body to hold myself together. During the dinner, the president of horticulture media did a small tribute to me and my work with the edible school gardens program. My friend who was sitting next to me seemed to sense I was in distress, because she pulled me into her arms, and I cried. As soon as I was able to, I left the event and drove home.

That Monday, I contacted my acupuncture friend, Phil McManus, and said, "I need help." Phil was so kind. Besides listening, giving me a treatment, and providing tissues as I cried the whole time, he stayed in contact with me every day and flooded me with positive encouragement.

After a bit of researching, I found a holistic doctor, and she diagnosed me with chronic fatigue. For the next couple of years, I threw myself into every natural health modality, desperately trying to get well, but I was so depleted, just struggling to put one foot in front of the other. In the end, it was my kinesiologist, Greg, who was brave enough to tell me that not only wasn't I getting better, I was deteriorating. Then he brought out what looked like a slide album, with each card having a different circle in it. He would point at a circle, and as I looked at it, he would check my arm strength. One of those cards indicated *Lyme*, and my arm went weak.

These are called 'Organisational Pattern Cards" (OPC) and may symbolically represent literally anything. They're typically used to create homoeopathic remedies with a radionics device, but my kinesiologist uses them to identify many types of imbalance at the physical, mental and emotional levels.

He said, "You have Lyme disease," and I said, 'What's Lyme?' But even though he explained the concept, it really meant nothing to me. There's a part of me that longs for these days of innocent, naïve bliss.

My doctor wouldn't believe him, until a few months later when I was too sick to attend a girlfriend's funeral and booked an emergency appointment. The doctor looked at me and said, "I think you have Lyme." I could have hit her. Why couldn't she have listened to me months ago?

She gave me a questionnaire with a list of symptoms. There are 144 of them, and they're always changing. Lyme is often called 'the great imitator,' as it takes on the properties of other illnesses.

From the Lyme Disease Association of Australia website: lymedisease.org.au

Lyme disease manifests as a multi-systemic illness that can result in symptoms *affecting random parts of the body including the muscles, joints, organs, brain, gastro-intestinal and neurological systems.*

Lyme disease is generally categorised into acute (early) and chronic*(late) stages of disease each with varying symptoms.* Most diagnosed cases in Australia have progressed to the late stage, *because there are no early intervention strategies in place to ensure appropriate treatment following tick bites.*

Symptoms in early-stage Lyme disease (close to the time of the bite) commonly include: flu-like symptoms, headaches, fever, swollen lymph nodes, fatigue, muscle aches and joint pain.

Symptoms in late stage Lyme disease *(extending to many months, or even years, following tick bite) often manifests as multi-systemic illness, which may include: gastro-intestinal problems, neurological problems, balance problems, chronic fatigue and random muscle and joint pain. Late-stage Lyme disease can be mild, moderate or severe and, if left untreated, cause severe disability or become fatal.*

Acute Lyme disease

There are many symptoms associated with acute (early signs of) Lyme disease. These signs are (but not limited to) flu-like symptoms with fevers, fatigue, swollen glands, sore throat, nausea and vomiting, headaches, stiff neck, light sensitivity and may include Bell's palsy and other neurological symptoms.

Symptoms

Lyme disease symptoms can appear quickly or gradually over time, and they're incredibly varied and can wax and wane. The first physical signs of Lyme infection are often flu-like symptoms – sore throat, headaches, congestion, stiffness, etc. – so many people, including doctors, dismiss the symptoms as the flu or the common cold.

During its nymph stage, a tick is only about the size of a period on a sentence. Many people are infected by nymph ticks, but don't suspect Lyme disease because they don't recall being bitten. In fact, 50% of people infected don't remember being bitten and ***less than 50% of people will get any over-emphasized rash****.*

Head, Face, Neck

- *Unexplained hair loss*
- *Headache, mild or severe, seizures*
- *Pressure in head, white matter lesions in brain (MRI)*
- *Twitching of facial or other muscles*
- *Facial paralysis (Bell's Palsy, Horner's syndrome)*
- *Tingling of nose, (tip of) tongue, cheek or facial flushing*
- *Stiff or painful neck*
- *Jaw pain or stiffness*
- *Dental problems*
- *Sore throat, clearing throat a lot, phlegm, hoarseness, runny nose*

Eyes/Vision

- *Double or blurry vision*
- *Increased floating spots*
- *Pain in eyes, or swelling around eyes*
- *Oversensitivity to light*
- *Flashing lights, peripheral waves or phantom images in corner of eyes*

Ears/Hearing

- *Decreased hearing in one or both ears, plugged ears*
- *Buzzing in ears*
- *Pain in ears, oversensitivity to sounds*
- *Ringing in one or both ears*

Digestive and Excretory Systems

- *Diarrhea*
- *Constipation*
- *Irritable bladder (trouble starting, stopping) or interstitial cystitis*
- *Upset stomach (nausea or pain) or GERD (gastroesophageal reflux disease)*

Musculoskeletal System

- *Bone pain, joint pain or swelling, carpal tunnel syndrome*
- *Stiffness of joints, back, neck, tennis elbow*
- *Muscle pain or cramps, (Fibromyalgia)*

Respiratory and Circulatory Systems

- *Shortness of breath, can't get full/satisfying breath, cough*
- *Chest pain or rib soreness*
- *Night sweats or unexplained chills*
- *Heart palpitations or extra beats*
- *Endocarditis, heart blockage*

Neurologic System

- *Tremors or unexplained shaking*
- *Burning or stabbing sensations in the body*
- *Fatigue, Chronic Fatigue Syndrome, weakness, peripheral neuropathy or partial paralysis*
- *Pressure in the head*
- *Numbness in body, tingling, pinpricks*
- *Poor balance, dizziness, difficulty walking*
- *Increased motion sickness*
- *Light-headedness, wooziness*

Psychological Well-being

- *Mood swings, irritability, bi-polar disorder*
- *Unusual depression*
- *Disorientation (getting or feeling lost)*
- *Feeling as if you are losing your mind*
- *Over-emotional reactions, crying easily*
- *Too much sleep, or insomnia*
- *Difficulty falling or staying asleep*
- *Narcolepsy, sleep apnoea*
- *Panic attacks, anxiety*

Mental Capability

- *Memory loss (short or long term)*
- *Confusion, difficulty thinking*

- *Difficulty with concentration or reading*
- *Going to the wrong place*
- *Speech difficulty (slurred or slow)*
- *Difficulty finding commonly used words*
- *Stammering speech*
- *Forgetting how to perform simple tasks*

Reproduction and Sexuality

- *Loss of sex drive*
- *Sexual dysfunction*
- *Unexplained menstrual pain, irregularity*
- *Unexplained breast pain, discharge*
- *Testicular or pelvic pain*

General Well-being

- *Phantom smells*
- *Unexplained weight gain or loss*
- *Extreme fatigue*
- *Swollen glands or lymph nodes*
- *Unexplained fevers (high or low grade)*
- *Continual infections (sinus, kidney, eye, etc.)*
- *Symptoms seem to change, come and go*
- *Pain migrates (moves) to different body parts*
- *Early on, experienced a "flu-like" illness, after which you've not since felt well*
- *Low body temperature*

- *Allergies or chemical sensitivities*
- *Increased effect from alcohol and possible worse hangover*

The doctor arranged for the first and only test we could do in Australia (Geelong, Victoria), for Lyme-related co-infections, so not actually Lyme disease but one of its co-infections caused from a tick, called Rickettsia. When the results came back, the doctor scrolled through them on her computer, showing me pages of information that meant nothing to me. She said, "I've never seen anyone with so many Rickettsia. You have five different types. No wonder you feel sick!"

I wasn't sure how to respond, as the doctor 's reaction was a mixture of engrossed, amused, and fascinated by my results. It was more like, "Oh, okay. Well, that is interesting, isn't it?"

She explained we would need further blood tests done in either Germany or the U.S.A. to see what other Lyme and co-infections I was dealing with. We had to send blood overseas as, again, Lyme isn't recognised in Australia. Most doctors know absolutely nothing about it or its symptoms or treatments, and when you're blessed enough to find a Lyme-literate doctor, they must refer to it as a Lyme-like illness! They can't say you have Lyme, even if you contacted the illness in this country. The survey questions you're asked are designed to get the answers the government wants, not the truth. For example: *Have you ever travelled overseas?* If you answer yes, your records will indicate you caught it overseas.

I went home and emailed my sister, just debriefing my brain as I always did with her. Anne-Maree wrote back and said she and her hubby, Peter, would pay for my blood tests in the U.S.A., so

I could get some answers. She wrote, *You've been sick for so long. We want to see you better.* God, I love my sister and her husband.

It then took a couple of months over the Christmas period to organise for my blood to be sent to the U.S.A to be tested. It was a long wait and expensive. My blood had a bigger holiday than I did.

CHAPTER 5

The Crying Time Bomb

My rock and foundation are my core support team that have been there for me since becoming 'mysteriously' unwell. They keep me together emotionally, sometimes phoning daily. They consist of: Jenny in Perth, Karen in Melbourne, Victoria, Fiona in Alice Springs, Costa in Sydney, NSW, and Anne-Maree in Victoria. Jenny and Fiona used to reside in the Noosa area, where I currently live.

I can't get through this on my own. Most friends and others don't know I'm unwell. Lyme people don't tend to look sick, unless you know them really well and can see it in their eyes and hear it in their speech, so it's easy to bluff my way through it. There are occasions when that filter dissolves instantly, like when a shop assistant innocently asks, "How are you today?" and I burst into tears.

The weird part is that the people I see regularly, such as at the post office and bank, have become my biggest supporters, extending much kindness and love to me over the years. I didn't know them to chat to before, except for pleasantries, but once I started crying and explaining my current health challenge, they were so compassionate. I feel like a crying time-bomb. I have no control over when I might start.

Longing to be well again, I'm meeting with incredibly supportive practitioners and so many generous, loving healers.

My typical day goes like this:

I wake up and put each foot on the floor before hobbling to the toilet while saying, "Ouch…ouch…ouch.". Fortunately, the pain doesn't last.

The yoga mat is by my bed, and I do a few stretches, a habit I've had for over twenty years, way before I was officially diagnosed. It gives me an indication of how my energy is. When I face plant, I know I don't have any, so I'll expect to spend the day in bed. If I'm going into the downward dog and fall on the ground crying and begging the universe to give me the strength to get me through this, I know I have to be gentle with myself and stay away from negative people or triggers. But of course, sometimes life isn't that simple.

From the yoga mat, I go into my favourite time of the day, when I feed and chat with the guinea pigs and chooks, collect greens while admiring and loving my abundant organic food gardens, and walk through my food forest to the lagoon, where I throw some sticks for Potcy. After I've had my fun, I go back inside to make breakfast, as I struggle to keep awake, my eyelids drooping. Then I prepare lunch before racing my daughter to the bus stop by 6.55am. By then, I'm struggling to function. Many times, my daughter offers to get herself breakfast and to the bus stop, but she would have to get up at 4.30 a.m. The least I can do is help at the start of her day.

At seven a.m., I literally crawl back into bed, the fatigue consuming every cell of my body, and fall into a rock-solid sleep for a couple of hours. These sleeps are always my deepest.

Then I get up for a couple of hours but never really achieve anything, as my brain fog is so bad. After my lunch, I'm back to bed for another couple of hours of sleep.

From two p.m. to four p.m. is usually my sweet spot of feeling 'normal' and being productive. This is when I try and get as much done as I can.

I need to be in bed by 8.00pm, otherwise my body will punish me severely with pain and exhaustion the next day for every minute I'm up past that time. Unfortunately, just because I'm tired, doesn't mean I sleep. The doctor has forbidden me from reading books about gardening and health while in bed. I must read something simple, where my brain isn't active. I never thought I would see the day where I would enjoy reading *Mills and Boon* books that consist of short love stories with predictable endings. Nights are always a surprise bundle of no sleep, hot sweats, feeling like thousands of bugs are crawling under my skin (as I punch myself for perceived relief), pain going through my body, and finding it hard to breathe. Sometimes I take a sleeping pill.

I know it's hard for Melika. Even though I try to not show how much Lyme is affecting me, she's the person who's around me the most and knows me so well. She worries and often tells me to go to bed, and she'll cook dinner. She's had to make sacrifices in her teenage years, because I can't stay up late to pick her up from any social events, and we live too far out of town for public transport. Her teachers are brilliant, and I wonder how often she goes to school and cries, not knowing if her mum will be well again, just as I don't know if I'm strong enough to get through it.

I was never going to go public with my Lyme disease. Many friends still don't know, as I can't bring myself to tell people without crying, so it's easier to say nothing's wrong and just withdraw from being in public and socialising. But mostly, it's because I feel like a failure. How can I no longer work? How do I not earn an income or participate in normal, everyday activities? Some days, I'm lucky to even know my own name.

But one morning, a voice in my head keeps saying, *You have to tell everyone.* I argue against it, but in the end, I text my daughters and tell them I'm going to announce it on Facebook. When everyone finds out their mother is sick, it will affect them.

I spend a long time writing and rewriting what to say and cry the whole time. Then I post it, and a huge sense of relief washes over me. Lots of people offer support and love. Some private message me to say they had Lyme, or thought they did. It's an enormously emotional day, but I feel lighter for it.

CHAPTER 6

Being Human

Because I haven't been able to work, I have no money, so I need to seek financial assistance from Centrelink, Human Services (Australia's welfare system). How they can call themselves human, as if it's their actual job to assist and care for Australian citizens, is truly beyond my comprehension.

Staff rarely treats me with any respect. I hate it, and you better believe how degrading it is for me to need government handouts to survive and be treated like I'm trying to rip off the system. I'm so tired, I have trouble following what these people are saying to me and can barely stay awake through their many, many interviews that are more like interrogations. There's nothing 'human' about the experience.

One staff nurse, an 'authority on people sickness,' is assessing me for my sickness benefit, and holds the pen to tick if I'm eligible for fortnightly payments. Even though the doctor has filled out medical certificate paperwork with all of my conditions, she has the overriding power.

Then she has the cheek to say to me, "You can't expect to sit around and do nothing and get paid for it!" I want to reply, "How many chronic fatigue (again, not allowed to say you have Lyme) people do you know who got sick from sitting around doing nothing?'" So disempowering. But I keep quiet, because I need that money to live.

I apply to access my superannuation. After providing all the paperwork and evidence from multiple doctors, naturopaths and therapists of treatments needed and the costs, my claim is rejected, because treatment for chronic fatigue is available through the public health system. What a joke!

The only thing several doctors wanted to give me before I found a holistic doctor, was anti-depressants. One doctor even refused to see me again, until I started on them. I said, "People commit suicide while taking anti-depressants," but their only response was that they monitor people. That's crap. I know they don't.

Centrelink constantly has me going back for mindless, pointless interviews. I'm on a medical certificate, meaning I'm not required to look for a job, but that doesn't stop them from telling me the hours I would need to work if I wasn't on a certificate. The main problem is that every time I get called back there, I have major panic attacks. My anxiety is already sky high, and this just adds another layer to it.

Sometimes my sister has to coach me via text, just so I can walk through the doors. How did my life turn out like this? What part of success makes a person rely on government assistance? It's not even enough to live on, let alone pay for medical expenses.

I also get family assistance benefit to help with costs associated with raising children. The staff are kind, supportive, and compassionate to my situation. My ex-husband (Melika's father), despite owning two retail shops that are sufficiently profitable to fund overseas trips and home renovations, contributes just $1.86 per week towards Melika's expenses. He's also able to creatively write off so many 'business' expenses, and thus claim he isn't earning enough to pay any more. Despite the unfairness around that, he also thought it amusing to belittle me when he heard I had had to resort to government support. Blows my mind why anyone would take pleasure in someone else's pain and fail to contribute fairly to his daughter's expenses.

The only way I've survived is Anne-Maree, who's been lending me money to pay for medical expenses, my daughter's needs, and anything else I don't have the money for. Otherwise, my daughter's life would look a lot different, and I would never be able to afford the costly treatments.

CHAPTER 7

The Healing Ritual

My symptoms at the moment consist of:

- major anxiety
- panic attacks, especially in public
- shakiness
- tingling in different parts of my body
- feeling like I have thousands of bugs crawling under my skin
- pain sometimes in knees, neck, or shoulder, or all at once
- painful feet to walk on at night and in the morning,
- nervy
- dry throat
- brain fog
- headaches
- shallow breathing
- terrible sleep no matter what techniques I use
- Hashimoto's disease (thyroid).

The crazy part is that I've spent ten years building a public profile with my Edible School Gardens programs, and also as a professional speaker and workshop presenter, so it's disheartening to no longer want anyone to recognise or speak to me.

I have an involved daily routine to help me alleviate the pain. There's my Infrared sauna that I use every day. It's a portable silver unit. I sit on a chair inside of it, and my head pops out the top. I also use a PowerTube that's a medical device for pain relief. It works on the skin and cycles through three stages that use high frequencies to provide relief. And then I detox in a bath with magnesium. In addition, I jump on a trampoline in my backyard for only a few minutes and do yoga stretches.

I have a healing group I go to on Mondays that has a smorgasbord of trained natural therapists to assist with healing. Practitioners include reiki, tarot, crystal healing, massage, reflexology, kinesiology, and cranial sacral. The sessions only cost twenty dollars for a thirty-minute session, and I usually have two or three each week, depending how I feel or what I need. I also see my doctor and receive acupuncture, Chinese medicine, and kinesiology during the month.

I have days when I wake up and feel good to the point where I believe I've 'nailed' this Lyme thing, and I'm cured … until I sit up in bed ready to start the day, and my body crashes again.

Nice thought, if only briefly.

CHAPTER 8

With A Little Help From My Friends

I love my organic property. The permaculture garden I've created attracts so many birds, including my favourites, kookaburras, king parrots, and lorikeets, as well as a kangaroo family. The roo mum loves to present her new joeys to me when they're old enough to pop their heads out of her pouch and comes up to me when I'm gardening. We always keep a respectful distance of approximately two metres, but I love how they trust me and understand this is their land and home, too. They never eat my vegetables, even in drought times. The father kangaroo is a different story, however, and I retreat to the house if I see him. He's way too big to trust.

My pool that I converted to a wetland has attracted so many happy frogs, and I love listening to them singing at night when the rain is coming down. The ducks swim in there, too. It feels good to have created so much with nature and attracting the wildlife. Their presence each day is like a meditation and gives me something to be grateful for.

No matter how tired I am, each morning and night I go to the edge of the lagoon and allow myself to just be. It's where I shed many tears and wonder how I'm going to get through this. Then I gently paddle up and down in my canoe. It's soothing, especially when the full moon is rising. I sit in the middle of the water and offer my list of wishes (demands) to the universe, pleading to make me strong enough to survive this. To make me whole and complete again.

Every month, I keep repeating my wishes. I'm not asking for much, just to return me to the person I once was, an energetic, positive, busy woman with successful projects. Someone who's celebrated for her experience, is loved by many, and feels happy, generous, and joyful.

But for now, I must drag this body around. I can barely do any gardening, a passion of mine I no longer have energy for. I'm lucky to have loyal permaculture friends who come on a regular basis to garden. They make me sit down and watch, which is harder for me than gardening. Sometimes, when the jobs mount up, the Permaculture Noosa Club arranges a working bee at my home, and permaculture friends, as well as people I've never met before, turn up and work hard while I just watch. I'm so very grateful.

My neighbour, Don, helps me maintain the inside and outside of my home. I make a list of jobs, and he does them for me. I know him and his wife, Fran, are always there to support me.

I put positive affirmations on my bathroom mirror and say them each time I'm in there, while trying really hard to believe them. My kinesiologist, Greg, helps release the sadness I feel by allowing me to let go of negative core beliefs (NCB) and replace them with positive core beliefs (PCB). I do find this powerful and useful. I can never get away with anything where he's concerned, either. If I try to pretend I have some other problem, as soon as he taps into me, he goes straight to where it actually is, which I'm indirectly grateful for, even though it brings me to tears.

I went to a Lyme support group in town, but they were all so negative and sick. I'd come there in a great mood, because I'd had some lovely treatments that day and was feeling good, and I'd been looking forward to meeting new people. But after a while, I felt guilty for feeling good and hated the down energy of the room. Life is hard enough without other people talking about how bad their life is.

I know support groups are an opportunity for release around like-minded people, but everyone seemed to want to wallow in their misery rather than using the time to come together and lift each other up. It's so important to have some type of support group, whether online, in person, or both, but I can't get weighed down too much by everyone else's pain, fear, sadness, and hopelessness. It's so important to find the right group of people for you, and I was proud of myself for not sticking around.

There are also good free podcasts and summits available. My favourite to listen to are health summits. *The Chronic Lyme Disease Summit 1*, produced by Dr Jay Davidson (*drjaydavidson.com/summits/*), was my first introduction to them, and it was life-saving!! For the first time, here was a series of educated, researched, health-focussed professionals who not only knew about Lyme but were also treating patients successfully without frying their bodies (hyperthermia) or other extreme drug treatments (long-term antibiotics). It's such a breath of fresh air, and there's hope…so much hope! There are positive, successful solutions out there! I finally feel like I've found people who truly understand this insidious disease and are there to support me.

People may say that your illness is a blessing; a gift that makes you become a better person. I don't agree with any of this. I loved my life before, BUT…I will say I've been blessed by the friendships and love I've experienced from my practitioners, new friends, and healers, some of whom were willing to do distance healing. Also, it fills me with a sense of peace to know that in several countries in the world, people are praying (in whatever belief they follow) for me.

It gives me so much strength to know that I do matter to someone.

CHAPTER 9

Leanne

My Chinese medicine/homeopathic practitioner, Leanne Levin, is intelligent and so passionate about getting me well. I knew her husband through permaculture before needing her talents. She's one sharp, switched-on practitioner.

We got on well, and while I had chronic fatigue, I still had some bookings to present garden talks that I'd committed to months earlier. Leanne came along and supported me. We even did one together. She was knowledgeable about food, so we spoke as a team. But what people didn't know was any time I faltered, Leanne took up the slack and kept me looking professional. When I gave her my Lyme results from the U.S.A., we sat on her chair together, and she showed me some solutions she would try. She was so supportive and loving.

In April 2015, Leanne died in a tragic accident, leaving behind two little girls and a distraught husband. She was much loved. Her husband phoned and asked me to be MC for her memorial service, and naturally I agreed. Then I got off the phone and burst into tears. How on earth was I going to do this? I had no energy at all, was in a constant state of brain fog, and explaining to a crowd how Leanne and I became friends, would mean publicly admitting I was sick.

The day arrived, and I had to distance myself from the crowd in order to hold my emotions together. I had two bottles of Australian Bush Flowers emergency essence near me. There were lots of people, plus a couple of video cameras recording the ceremony for her daughters to watch when they were older. None of those things made me nervous. Beside me was her family, sitting to the left of the podium. I didn't look their way, but I could hear Leanne's mother's deep, heart-wrenching sobs.

A couple of times at the beginning I teared up, but I looked to heaven and asked Leanne to give me strength, and I continued. Then when her husband spoke, the rawness of his pure love for his wife, the mother of their daughters, with so much personal detail...it just broke my heart. Everybody was crying. Tears flooded down my face, but I pulled myself together to make a closing statement honouring Leanne and her family and friends. It was such a beautiful ceremony.

The final song started, so I had said my goodbyes and turned to move away, when someone came up and hugged me. I think it was her brother. I broke down. I'd held those tears in all week. Many people, including her parents, thanked me for a beautiful service. I was so relieved I'd done Leanne and her family proud.

I was honoured to be invited to their home with their families for lunch following the ceremony. And although this event made me sick for many weeks afterward, forcing me to pull on already-worn out, non-existent adrenals, it was one of the most uplifting days of my life. While grieving Leanne's death and desperately wishing she were still here, I was so honoured to be trusted by her families to represent them in front of her friends and peers, and to be able to personally honour my girlfriend at her passing. I miss you, Leanne.

CHAPTER 10

The Wave Of The Future

September 2015

I'm taking so many supplements, vitamins, potions, and treatments, but I don't seem to be making any progress. I need to search out more progressive/radical practitioners by thinking outside of the box. At night I'm waking with sweat running down my stomach and heat purges radiating through my body. I need some sleep.

I feel blessed to find Rasunah, who owns an online business with natural and health products. She's a wealth of wisdom, is supportive, and has lots of alternative, natural therapies, while also encouraging people to do coffee enemas. Not to get too personal, but I've never even drunk coffee, as I hate the smell, and now I have to stick it up my butt. OMG. The things you do in the quest for wellness.

In addition to the other therapies I mentioned, through Rasunah's suggestions, I'm also on the Pulsed Electromagnetic field therapy (PEMF), using a Biomat (an infrared sauna and negative ions crystal mat), and have purchased a trampoline rebounder lymphasizer. (A definition for all of these therapies is provided at the back of this book.) Rasunah is my latest super support woman. She just knows what I need.

However, things don't go well with my first coffee enema. I get myself all set up on the outdoor deck, so I can relax and get some sunshine on my skin at the same time. I have towels to lie on and some relaxing music. People say enemas are a time to meditate and relax, and I'm all set up for it. I have my instructions next to me and a timer set for fifteen minutes.

Well, my experience is the polar opposite of relaxing. After a few minutes, the container holding the coffee liquid is empty, and I can only assume it's sloshing around in my liver and colon somewhere. Suddenly, I can't hold it in. There's an enormous sense that it's all going south.

I try to make my way to the toilet a mere ten metres away, shuffling through the house with a towel between my legs. When I finally get to the bathroom, I make one disgusting mess as my bowels explode. I'm sweating profusely, I feel like I'm going to faint, and I nearly pass out. I lie on the cold tiles, overheated, exhausted and upset. How did my life end up like shit?

I stay on the floor for a long time before I recover enough to start cleaning up. Then I shower in tears. But this taught me a valuable lesson. I learned I really need to pay attention to instructions and not have the bucket higher than 30–40 cms (12–16 inches), and from talking to others, I found out it's okay to start slowly and not hold the liquid in for the full fifteen minutes. I can start with only five minutes and increase each time. Also, and this can't be stressed enough, I need to always do the enema next to the toilet.

I really feel like crap. I used to have so much fun in my life and be so vibrant, energetic, and happy. Now I'm fatigued all the time.

CHAPTER 11

What's The Frequency?

October 2015

I'm now going to a SCIO bioresonance device therapist. Wow! Everyone should do this! The therapist puts special straps around my head, wrist and ankles that connect back to the computer. The procedure doesn't hurt. I don't feel anything. In fact, I have a hard time staying awake, as my first appointment is for more than ninety minutes. Our bodies are made up of a distinctive electromagnetic signature within every cell, emotion, meridian, and organ, and this machine taps into your whole body to find out what's stressing it the most, whether it's emotionally, physically, on a cellular level, or if you have parasites. All of that yummy info.

And it's doing a treatment on me at the same time, with its frequency. It even tests products/supplements to figure out if my body wants them. The medicine of the future. I'm so impressed. It even knows my inner, secret thoughts (fears) and comes up with a positive statement for me to practise every day. *I AM ENOUGH!* Right, machine. You'll have a hard time trying to convince me I'm nothing. From now on, I'm somebody. *I am Enough.*

In addition, she also gives me homeopathic tablets that I take every morning and night.

Word seems to have got out that I'm curing myself naturally, and other people who have Lyme have started contacting me. Considering how few people I told, I'm surprised. Some were referred by my healing practitioners and others through my permaculture friends. I catch up with one person for a cuppa or lunch each week, since that's as much as I can manage. Then I get too sick to leave the house for a couple of weeks and don't see anyone, which adds to my list of things to do. But in the midst of my misery, I have a light bulb moment. I'll get all of these people together as a positive, natural Lyme support group!

When I inform them of my idea, everyone loves it, and our small group is born. It's so good to meet others on the same path, with the same mindset of wellness and support. We're all like scientists, researching constantly, and each month we report back to the group what we've discovered or new practitioners we've seen that were good/bad/had no idea, plus the latest informative book, YouTube, summit, etc.

It's really fast-tracked our journey, and we lament that it's a crime against humanity that it's up to us to do our own research. We're lucky to have doctors on the Sunshine Coast trained in treating Lyme, especially with supplements. Excuse me, I mean a 'Lyme-like illness.'

It's been fantastic and so important to have a group of Lyme friends who truly understand what I'm going through. Brit, especially, is there for me when I'm swallowed up by a dark cave of depression and my dark night of the sad soul. She keeps an eye on me all day and sends positive messages. Brit and I knew each other through work in what we call our 'previous life.' Like me, she had got a tick bite years earlier, and we were functioning fine, but we both went through highly stressful situations that lowered our immunity and triggered the Lyme response. It helps with supporting each other, because we know what we've lost, professionally, physically, socially, and in our personalities, though this illness. Only someone who's going through the same experience can really understand where I'm at and know what to say. If I voice what I'm thinking to my Anne-Maree, it will scare her, and anyway, she's too far away to just drop in. Though she always says she and her husband will come any time to help, and I know she means it.

There are six of us in my Lyme group, which is a perfect number. This size means we can stay intimate and express exactly what we're feeling, with total support and without judgment. We share our stories and exchange information. I love this group of women who have so much wisdom to share, and we just seem like a bunch of friends catching up for lunch. The problem with Lyme is that you don't look unwell, and therefore you can be treated or judged harshly by unknowing people who are unaware of your inability to return to work or operate at full capacity. Only we can see who isn't coping well that day and are there to help them through difficult times.

CHAPTER 12

Everything Is All Right

I wake up at 5:30 a.m. to get Melika organised and get her to the bus stop for school. Sometimes I'm late and have to chase the bus, or even worse, drive her all the way into town. My body is so tired. How did my life end up like this? No energy, no projects, no fun, no adventures, and no end date to when I'll be well again. Will I ever get better??? The hardest part is that friends have walked away from me in my greatest time of need or don't invite me to events anymore. They don't want me around, as I can't drink alcohol and have limited energy, so I'm not the life of the party. I'm no longer the energetic, positive powerhouse I once was. I miss me.

From my diary:

> *Why did my life jack-knife?*
>
> *Why has my life turned to shit?*
>
> *I used to have an open door to visitors, but now I'm too tired to tolerate people staying.*
>
> *I rarely hear from my good friends.*

I hate Lyme disease. I don't want to live a life not worth living. I have no fun, I have no joy, and where have all my friends gone? I've been dumped faster than hot shit.

I hate having a body that feels so tired and shaky.

I want to experience life. I want to be part of life. LIVING—not fucking wondering if I'm just better off dying.

I want someone to wrap their arms around me and hold me tight and tell me that EVERYTHING is going to be all right. I'm so scared.

I can't and don't want to keep doing this on my own. Loneliness is no sainthood. What has happened to this world? What happened to community and caring and support?

I want to live a LIFE, not be controlled by taking medicines and doing treatments (though grateful to have them) all day.

I just want someone to HOLD, to tell me I'LL BE OK!!! And take some of my troubles away. PLEASE. I can't do this on my own anymore. I don't want to.

I visit my naturopath with symptoms of brain fog and chronic fatigue. I'm just sooo tired, emotional, and depressed. I also have tinnitus, insomnia, and a shaky nervous system We do some emotional clearing and work on taking my NCBs and turning them into PCBs.

I'm taking so many supplements every day to try and rebuild my body and kill the unwelcome. I've listed them below in a general way, so you can get some idea of where my quest for wellness has taken me. *[This list is deliberately vague, as every body is unique and will have different requirements. Disclaimer: this isn't medical advice.]*

With Each Meal:	**Waking**	**Before Every Meal**
Beyond Balance syrup drops	Homeopathic tabs	Vitamin C
Tox-ease GL. Lymph-support	General Salt tissues tabs	Bowel Restore (15-30 minutes before meal)
IMN-V-III.	Thyroid tab.	

Breakfast	**Lunch**	**Dinner**
Veg Digestive Enzymes	Veg Digestive Enzymes	Veg Digestive Enzymes
AdrenoTone	AdrenoTone	AdrenoTone
D3	SamE	D3 sprays
Zinc	Zinc	Zinc
Hydrozyme	Chromium	PRL Max B ND drops
SamE	Bilberry	Chromium
Chromium	Curcumin	Women's essentials
Women's essential vitamins	Hydrozyme	Hydrozyme
Max vitamin B	Xenostat thyroid	Macula saffron
G tox detox	Biohawk ginger/pine	Billberry
Biohawk ginger/pine	Magnesium	G tox detox
Magnesium	Lemon balm drops	Magnesium
Lemon balm drops		Biohawk ginger/pine with pepper

Mid-Afternoon	**Before Bed**
5htp. Gabba	Gabba
	5htp.
	Melatonin
	Probiotic
	Homeopathic tabs

I think because I don't know the future, my mind is in a tug-of-war. Do I just punish my body and try to achieve some fun and purpose in my life while continuing to do endless treatments, or do I just give up? It's so hard to think anything positive. I know compared to most Lyme people, I don't have many symptoms, but I don't like being sick, I don't like not living, and I don't like spending most of my days and nights exhausted and alone. This isn't *living*.

Fuck, fuck, fuck. I hate this.

CHAPTER 13

Ice Cold

I have a tenant living in the detached cabin on my property. His car isn't working, and it's in another town, so I offer him a lift to catch up with his girlfriend. I'm a bit confused by what he's saying, but I'm aware he's under a lot of stress lately. He's been doing some weird stuff, and I even found him asleep in his car at six a.m. one morning when he should have been at work.

I drop him at the shops and continue on, and I'm collecting cardboard for the garden from the back of an office building, when his girlfriend pulls up alone and says, "Leonie, I need to talk to you."

Mystified, I say, "Sure."

She says, "Leonie, have you any idea what's happening in your cabin? What my boyfriend is doing?"

Innocently, I confess that I don't.

Then she drops the bombshell: "He's making ice (a drug) and dealing it."

And it gets worse. She tells me she has a domestic violence order (DVO) against him, and his previous girlfriend had one, too. As I wait for the information, I'm starting to form some kind of pathway in my brain, I just focus on her and ask if she's okay.

She advises me to be careful, and I ask her to not let him know I'm aware of what he's doing, so I can work out what action I'll take.

I get in my car and drive in a complete shocked daze, just saying, with a sense of doom, "Oh fuck … Oh fuck." I have no idea what to do. I have no experience with people on ice. I only know what the TV tells me, and that is frightening.

I talk to some people and realise this is a major problem. My friend Tansy, being ex-real estate, is up to date on the signs of ice. It all falls into place in my mind, and it's not positive. Now I understand why the water pump was going on and off all the time and why he always sprayed his unit with aftershave. It was to cover up the smell. I'm so naïve.

The next morning, his girlfriend visits. They have an argument, and she drives off angry and fast. He goes back inside his unit, and I hear the water pump going on and off, indicating he's up to something in the drug-making process. I so wish I didn't have to deal with this.

I call the police after I'm sure of what he's doing, and, if can you believe this…they're NOT interested!! WTF? But I'm not getting off the phone, as I need help to deal with the situation. They ask his name, and when I tell them, that's when they become interested. They've been looking to serve him a DVO notice but didn't have a current address. Police finally arrive hours later, with me a nervous, depleted woman. They speak to him at length and then leave … without him! He's still on my property! OMG, what am I going to do?

Friends have been trying to get Melika and me to find another place to stay, but I won't leave my animals. I phone my tenant and pretend I know nothing. I just say, "Why were the police here? I'm upset. As a single mum, I don't want police showing up. It looks bad to the neighbourhood." He tells me about being in trouble but offers no details, and then he says he would never want to upset me or worsen my health. I tell him he must leave, and, I can't believe my luck when he agrees to move out later in the week.

That week before he leaves is enormously stressful. I jump at each noise and lock my daughter in the house every time I go out to the animals. When he finally goes, I feel awful for not saying goodbye. I was so lucky he's only ever been a gentleman to me, and I feel no anger towards him, although I'm nervous about walking into the cabin to see what damage there is. But he's cleaned it beautifully. There are just some burn marks on the kitchen bench, and he's left a full-page letter to me wishing me well and thanking me for being such a good landlady. Yeah, I bet. He's just thankful I was so ignorant. The one saving grace was that he only used the unit for cooking and not for dealing. I guess you need to be thankful for the little things.

CHAPTER 14

Sound Alchemy

What a day! After much encouragement by some spiritual friends, I have a private healing session with Julian from Sound Alchemy, who's visiting from Perth and is doing ancient/indigenous healing with sound. He uses the crystal didgeridoo, traditional didgeridoo, crystal bowls, a rain stick, and other indigenous musical instruments.

I lie on the floor with my eyes shut, and he does a meditation over me before playing the different instruments and moving them along my body. The feeling is incredible. Vibrations go through every layer of my body. It's euphoric. Afterwards, I'm on a natural high. I have NO PAIN or any symptoms, and my body is oozing with energy. Julian warns me to be quiet all day to allow the healing to settle into my body.

I can't believe how good I feel. The world is bright and beautiful, and everything is possible. I don't even have heat purges, and I'm not sweating. I feel like I could do anything. I never thought I would feel like this again. I'm whole and complete. It's like I'm in love. New, juicy love.

Though the effects only last a couple of days, it's made a huge impact on my determination to beat this disease and be fully alive once more. I feel blessed to have been given an insight into wholeness, health, joy, and love again, but then there's the low of being back to fatigue, pain, endless supplements, detox routines, and appointments. And back to mattress island! Sleep land. I need a break from my life. I'm so strict with my routines but never get everything done with all of the sleeps. I also need to deal with my emotions. I try Quantum Healing Hypnosis Technique (QHHT). It's interesting to go back into some previous lives and find the message in them. I'm not sure how it's going to help me right now, but I know the messages are relevant.

CHAPTER 15

Proud Mom

I do as much as I can for Melika to support her though her assignments and leading up to exams. She's under so much stress to achieve at a high level and is working hard. I'm pushing myself to help, as I want to be there for her, so I don't show the toll it's taking on me.

The pressure of year 12, the final year of high school in Australia, is massive. She has a huge day at school and then must deal with me when she comes home. Sometimes she has to watch over me or listen to me moan in pain as I get into bed. I try to never let her hear me cry, though. It's not fair to offload all of my pain and grief onto my children. I feel guilty and sad that I can't be the mother I want to be for both of my girls. So often, I can't even remember what they've done or are doing, and I'm always asking them the names of their friends, as I don't retain that information.

They rarely have friends come over, which upsets me, as our home was meant to be full of friends and family. But the truth is, I'm relieved. I can't manage it for lots of reasons. My brain fog is so bad. One day I drove off and realised I had no idea where I was going and had to look for hints in the car. What am I wearing?

What's on the passenger seat? In my basket? Do I have a to-do list? I'm sitting there piecing together clues. It's scary. Many times I have no idea where I am or what I'm meant to be doing.

At last, Melika finishes her year 12 exams, and we have her graduation ceremony at school. I'm feeling so unwell. My stomach is cramping, bloated, and painful, and I'm so tired. I'm sitting in the audience when they announce the students with the top marks for year 12. My daughter is named top of two subjects, and people start clapping, as most students win only one. And when they continue announcing the next four subjects, I'm thrilled to discover she's topped the class with six subjects in all. She's done it!

I'm absolutely beside myself, with pride bursting out of my chest. I love this girl so much. I want to run up to the podium and kiss her and hug her and tell the whole audience what an amazing person she is. I also want to hug her teachers, thank them and say, "WE DID IT!" I'm fist-pumping the air, I'm so happy. Everyone knows I'm the mother of this incredible student. That she's my flesh and blood.

Then they announce the top three students for the year. I warn the guy next to me that I may get excited again. After they announce third and second, I know she's number one. Yes! Dux of the school! I nearly kiss the man. My hands are dancing in the air. I'M SO PROUD. Melika deserves Dux. She's worked diligently for this honour.

Once the ceremony is over, I manage to thank some of her teachers but need to go home for a sleep. I feel like shit! The excitement has given my adrenals a good squeeze, and they're not happy. I'm emotionally shaky and lack any vitality. There's still a celebration that evening, and I need to nap in order to get through it. At home, I crawl into bed, and the pain increases tenfold throughout my whole body, which often happens when I lie down. I feel like I want to vomit.

After a restful sleep, I do a sound bowl meditation. I need to remain calm for Melika's graduation dinner tonight and gather strength, as my ex-husband will be seated next to me.

Once I'm there and settled, the awkwardness is palpable. I feel sorry for the other people at our table who sense the negative vibe between us. Melika keeps coming and checking on me and fussing, worried they haven't given me the right food, since I can't eat grain or dairy. She tells me it's okay if I need to leave, but I must stay long enough to see her get presented. I'm so glad I did. It was another proud moment.

When I finally get home to bed, I know it will take me days to recover. For a long time, I'll continue to tell everyone how my daughter was DUX of the school. I'm such a proud mum.

Melika receives her external exam results in December. She gets a Queensland OP1 (99%), which is the highest score possible. She did it! All of those endless days and nights studying, and the discipline to use every minute wisely, have been rewarded. My heart explodes with love, happiness, and pride. I feel so blessed to be her mum. I want to tell the whole world but will wait a day or two to let Melika have her glory first. I don't know how she did it, coming home to a sick mum and still staying on task, but I thank goodness she did.

CHAPTER 16

I'll Be Home For Christmas

It's early December 2015, and I have to start planning for my trip to my hometown for Christmas. Just thinking about it makes me exhausted. I've cancelled all social events—not that I had a full social calendar anyway—but I must try to reduce my anxiety and stress levels. I also have to find friends to look after Potcy, the chooks, and the guinea pigs.

Melika and I fly to Melbourne from the Sunshine Coast. Karen, my best friend from my hometown of Bendigo, meets us at the airport, and we drive to her home at Kilmore for a quick stop before going on to Bendigo to stay with Anne-Maree and Peter. I'm so thankful Peter has already checked what food I can eat and has done a shop for me. He'll also do the cooking for us. I'll be nourished and nurtured here, which is something I crave and desperately need. And sure enough, when we get there, we're welcomed with a warm, healthy curry.

The next day, we visit my mother, and her opening comment is, "You look awful!" It immediately distresses me. Melika quickly comes to my defence and says, "Mum's looking good at the moment," but my mother has to say, "You're looking old, too." I want to say *I haven't exactly been living the dream life.* But there's no point. I realise she has no understanding of the true nature of my illness and has no interest in hearing how I've been trying to get well. I feel upset. I'm so hurt that my own mother hasn't shown me support and doesn't realise how her comments upset me. Why have I bothered to come home?

My inner child has been wounded again. I know she disapproves of me not taking antibiotics, but I'm the one in the trenches, constantly researching the latest methods to be fully well again. I still refuse to take drugs, as my Lyme is chronic, not acute. I got my tick bite sixteen years ago, and although I used to get really tired, I'd been easily able to function as if I was really healthy, fit and strong … until I went through continuous stress, and my immunity dropped. Then Lyme had a chance to take over and became stronger than my immunity. My gut feeling is that I need to rebuild my body naturally and to seek out those who know how to treat it naturally.

We visit my old neighbours, Maxie and Des. I grew up with their children, and they're excited to see us. They're so positive and joyful. I spend the next few days catching up with friends, and it really is great to see them again. Bendigo is in drought, and there's no green. I'm missing the subtropics and abundant gardens where I live, so I go for a walk in the forest near my sister's house to get a touch of nature. I collect white stones in the forest and make love hearts to bring a smile to whoever passes by.

Christmas Day arrives. My brother, Michael, brings Melika home. She went out with her cousin, Mia, the night before, so she's a bit sluggish. Michael and I have a good catch-up sitting at the kitchen table, surrounded by all of my supplements, with my PowerTube beeping every seven minutes as it goes through its cycles.

I'm supposed to collect Mum to drop her at church and then collect her afterwards, but I can barely keep my eyes open while I'm driving her there, and the pain is increasing. I must get to bed ASAP, so I organise another brother to collect her.

Most of the family is gathered together, which consists of my two sisters, three brothers, five nieces and nephews with their partners, and Mum. As the preparations continue, it all gets overwhelming for me. I start crying and go to Anne-Maree. Melika is concerned. I can't cope with so much at once.

A long table is set for lunch, and I sit in the middle, but I find it quite interesting that no one is sitting next to me. I haven't been home for years, and I'm leaving in a couple of hours, yet not one member of my family will get near me. I think they're scared to get too close. Do they think I'm dying? Are they afraid to talk to me? But eventually the table fills, and people sit next to me, so I feel a little better. Afterward, we open presents. I've brought games for everyone all centred around the theme 'you need to have fun and joy in your life.'

My sister, Trish, has the car ready to drive us to the airport, which is two hours away. I'm crying again. I'm so scared. I don't know what's going to happen with this Lyme thing, and I don't want to leave my family. I want their support, but Queensland is my true home now. I can't stay here.

I hug everyone goodbye. Mia, my niece and godchild, walks me to the car while promising she will visit and help me. Anne-Maree, of course, is there, too, and is my constant rock throughout this.

I sleep in the car. At Melbourne airport, we phone Fedora, who's in England studying, to wish her Happy Christmas. She sounds homesick.

CHAPTER 17

Home Again

So good to be home and be by my lagoon again with my pets and nature friends. I sit in my canoe and just enjoy the peace and quiet. I love it here. I love being able to pick fresh food every day and collect the eggs (when the chooks feel up to it). I love sitting on my deck upstairs with the kookaburras and magpies joining me, and looking out over my property, just smiling and knowing that everything will be okay.

My friend Andrew takes me out for lunch for my birthday. I'm fifty-two. I love being at a restaurant and salivate over every mouthful of quality food. I don't stress about what I order (within reason), and just thoroughly enjoy the beautiful food, service, company and normality. Melika cooks me dinner, but I'm too tired to enjoy it.

For days I've had a terrible headache, and it's painful to lift my head. The osteopath adjusts my spine and says it will take a couple of days before I feel any improvements. That night I'm in *so much pain* all along my forehead and temples, and the base of my skull feels like a brick is about to crush my neck. I send a message to my osteopath, and she tells me to get to a doctor. Unfortunately, all of my doctors and therapists are on Christmas holidays, so I'm forced to see the one who's available. He notes I have a fever and orders some blood tests but tells me he thinks I may have viral meningitis and to go Emergency at the hospital if I get worse. When I leave, I walk lightly to soften the pain that shoots up my spine with every step. I feel sick, I have a fever and pain in my head, and I can't cope with any light.

I tell Melika I'm going to bed with my mobile phone, even though I hate having EMF in my room, but this is an exception. She cancels her work and other commitments to stay home with me. I last the night but wake Melika in the morning to take me to hospital. I'm holding my head that feels as heavy as a boulder and like it's going to explode.

At the hospital, they roll their eyes about Lyme. I go onto an IV drip, and Melika keeps getting me more blankets, as I'm freezing, and catches my vomit in a cup thing. She's a fabulous nurse.

I hate being here. The doctor isn't friendly. I want to get out, so I eventually tell them that the pain is reducing. I'm allowed to leave later that day, even though the doctor knows I'm lying and advises me to come back if I get worse. At least he gives me some vomiting and pain reduction drugs to help.

I go straight home and into bed. After I nap, I feel only marginally better. The vomiting hangs around for another week or so, but each day the pain reduces, and I'm slowly moving around more and eating again. When my doctors and health practitioners return from holidays and I tell them what happened, they all inform me straight away it's the Lyme. My body couldn't cope with being at the airport and on the plane with radiation everywhere, plus all of the chemicals/pesticides sprayed in airports and planes. I take weeks to recover, and I can't stand for long. I take a lot of naps, but night-time sleeping seems optional. I'm writing for a gardening magazine and struggle to make sense of my words. I finally get it done but can't take the photos, as I'm unable to stand upright long enough to organise them. Also, I have tinnitus in my ears again.

CHAPTER 18

Positive Core Beliefs

February, 2016

There's no point telling people when I'm not well, as I've been sick too long, and they've lost interest. I'm now going to pretend my life and health are just fine! As Norman Doidge, MD, psychiatrist and author of *The Brain That Changes Itself* says, "Stop wasting what little energy you have to express distress to those that can't help you." For me, it's Karen, Jen, Tracey (a friend from Toastmasters), Anne-Maree, Fiona, my neighbours Don and Fran, and my Lyme friends. There's also Penny, who's always here gardening for me.

I want to live a life again. I sometimes go to the local spiritualist church just as a place to hang out. It's escapism, really. I find it uplifting, but I cry when they start singing songs like "You Are Not Alone," which make me feel exactly that. But to prove me wrong, someone always holds my hand and gives me comfort as I cry.

In a fortnight, Melika will fly to Melbourne to start university. I will miss her so much. We've become really close over the last few years, but to be honest, I'm frightened to be on my own. What if something happens, and there's no one here to get me to hospital or call an ambulance? I'm already crying from the thought of her not being around. I never thought I would struggle with empty nest syndrome, but I'm a mess.

For her sake, I manage to pull myself together. One night when she arrives home, she gives me a huge hug, sobs and says, "Mum, I'm going to miss you so much." I hold myself together. I want to cry and let her know how much I'm going to miss her, too, but I don't want to make it harder for her to leave. I would never, ever want her to forego university to babysit me.

She flies out on 19 February 2016. I think my heart is going to break. Every time I walk past her bedroom, I start crying again. She's left a letter for me on the table, but I don't open it until hours later. It's so beautiful. She writes about how much she loves me and what a positive influence I've been to her. This is what keeps me going. I must be a good role model for my girls. I have to be strong for them and not just throw in the towel, but sometimes it's so hard.

I see my kinesiologist, Greg, for support again, to bring the negative core beliefs to the surface and replace them with positive ones. He reminds me that I need to keep repeating the NCBs until the PCBs are stronger and become the new norm. It's a powerful process.

This is my NCB:

My reality is that my life lacks joy. There's a sense of fatigue, a loss of purpose, and a lack of inspiration. I feel anger, depression, vengefulness, jealousy, broken-heartedness, and my self-esteem has been eroded. I'm left with a sense of fiery anger that's contained within and damages me at the biological level.

This is my PCB:

I have what's required to ***allow myself to let go*** *of my attachments to the past and the accompanying disruptive energies. With this process, I enable my deeper purpose to be revealed to me, heal my heart, and manifest real JOY in my Life.*

I've discovered the Asyra bioenergetic machine/treatment, another type of biofeedback computer system. It's a similar operation to the SCIO machine, but it has more programs running in the computer and therefore is able to detect more dis-ease/stress/imbalance in the body. Wow! Talk about the medicine of the future!

You hold onto brass rods that are connected to a computer system, and it works out what's stressing your body the most in that moment, so even if you have Lyme, your biggest stress can be heavy metals or parasites, and therefore you need to deal with those particular problems first. It also tells you which Lyme co-infections are active, as well as heaps of other information. And while you're being tested, it's working on fixing you.

Then the practitioner makes homeopathic drops with the frequency that you require, according to the results on the machine. The priority for me is to treat heavy metals first, then toxins and chemicals, followed by viruses, including Epstein Barr. Lyme co-infections are dealt with after the body is cleaner.

I can barely stay awake on the drive home. Thank goodness another Lyme friend, Carol, drove me, as it's about two hours each way and zaps my energy for days.

I meet a couple that make the Brown's gas machine. In brief, Brown's gas forms when an electric current is run through water, which results in the splitting of the water molecules and allows the hydrogen and oxygen to act independently of each other. The water becomes electrically expanded, absorbs electrons, and then expands to a gaseous state that's not steam or water vapor.

So I go to their home and try it on my chest. I don't notice any difference at first and maintain my usual tiredness, but that night I go to a friend's birthday party, one of the rare social events I do attend, and feel energetic. Everyone keeps telling me how good I look, and I do feel it, at least for a couple of hours before it's time to sleep. I'm going to buy one of these machines and hope it helps. Honestly, I'll try anything if I think it's going to make me better. I want to live life again. Please.

CHAPTER 19

So Close

In 2016, Senator John Madigan pushed successfully to have a senate enquiry into Lyme disease in Australia. There is total and complete ignorance around the topic. The government and the medical system are in denial, for whatever reason.

As I encountered time and again through questionnaires and seeing many doctors, there's a stubborn adherence to the belief that Australia is immune to Lyme disease, and people only get it from being overseas.

There were 1,268 submissions to the Australian Government, which was just the number of Lyme-affected people or organisations that had that the energy or faith to respond. It certainly doesn't represent the true thousands, perhaps tens of thousands, of Australian people who are suffering with Lyme disease, diagnosed or undiagnosed. All of the submissions are available to read online. You can find them at: *aph.gov.au* under *Parliamentary Business*.

I read a couple of hundred submissions over several months. There's so much pain, sickness. and desperation. It's truly heartbreaking. I did send in mine, which included my entire Lyme journey, my frustration with trying to convince doctors of my condition, and the many therapies I'd undertaken, along with the substantial cost involved.

Unfortunately, due to an election, the inquiry never resulted in any assistance or recognition for Lyme patients. With the kind of response they received, how could the government not react favourably to help us?

Despite it not coming to fruition, I want to thank Senator John Madigan for his support with this inquiry and being a strong voice on our behalf.

CHAPTER 20

Not In This Country

March 2016

I go to the doctor, as I haven't slept all night due to the pain in my foot. She organises an ultrasound that doesn't find anything. My health isn't improving, my thyroid is declining, and I feel tired all day, every day. It's hard to be positive when I feel like shit, and I'm lucky to even pull some weeds out of my garden.

To top it off, Centrelink won't accept any more medical certificates from the doctor, as apparently no one can be sick longer than two years, so they're forcing me back to work. My doctor says I must fight Centrelink, as I'll only get sicker again if I try to push my body.

But who would employ me anyway? My brain fog is so bad, I'm too incapable of following any instructions. I would love to be back at work fulltime. I've worked all my life. I love working. I'm not some dole bludger. I don't need this extra stress.

I do as the doctor says and talk to the Federal MP's PA about my problem. We speak at length, and she's so understanding, it's hard for me not to cry. She gives me the tools to handle the interview, including what to do when they tell you to sign a piece of paper saying you *will* work the set hours, and you're actively looking for work.

I front up for my interview at the employment agency. When my interviewer puts several sheets of paper in front of me and tells me to sign them, I put the pressure/responsibility back on her and say, "I can't guarantee I can work these hours, so *you* need to guarantee to the employer that I can, because I can't." Wow. She doesn't like that.

The scene is repeated a couple of times, before she accuses me of raising my voice at her (I didn't, I just spoke firmly), and she brings in the manager to deal with me. Perfect. Not knowing what else to do, they decide I have a 'mental disability' and book me to see their psychologist. I'm not sure where she got her training, but the interview is appalling and so degrading, and she's just lucky I'm not having a bad day, because she deserves some abuse for belittling me.

First, she says, "Not much on your resume. You haven't done much in your life." And I think, *What have you done, sweetheart? Sit behind a desk and judge people all your life? Have you published a book, a DVD, and run your own business like I have?* Of course, I don't say that out loud. She continues with, "You left school at year 11. What marks did you get? C? D?" How rude! Back in my school days, finishing year 12 wasn't required to get a job, and how dare she assume I had low intelligence.

I wish I was quick enough to come back with something equally extreme, but my brain won't cooperate. Seeing that this interview isn't addressing the issue, and she still has a pile of pages in front of her, apparently about me, I ask, "Do you know why I'm here?" When she says she doesn't, I tell her I have Lyme disease, to which she gives the standard reply, "It's not in this country." Then she becomes the expert and tells me it's not curable. In the end, the manager is invited back in, and they agree I have a mental disability!

Next, I have an appointment with a different psychologist to jump through more hoops. This one is equally disrespectful and rude. Oh, Lord, give me strength! Is it any wonder mental disability is on the rise if this is the disrespect shown to someone who's worked all her life?

I hate depending on the small payments, and the way I'm treated brings out the worst in me personally, as I try to protect myself. My symptoms always get worse when I'm dealing with Centrelink. The anxiety and depression can get really bad, but I refuse to give them the pleasure of watching me break down in front of them. I leave that for when I get inside my car.

CHAPTER 21

A Difficult Decision

April 2016

I can't cope with the financial stress any longer. I hate owing my sister so much money. Every month, she helps me pay for all of my treatments, and my 'health debt' has accumulated. There are other treatments that I want to try, but they're expensive, and I can't expect her to be a bottomless pit of money for me. She even offered to send me to Germany for their radical heat treatment, but I said that probably wouldn't work for me anyway. Centrelink stresses me so much. I'm never going to get well while I'm dealing with them and the unnecessary stress they inflict on me with their lack of compassion and understanding.

So, I decide to sell my beautiful, organic property that I love so much. It's a difficult decision and breaks my heart, but I feel I have no other choice, as I can't see any time soon when I could do enough work to just pay the bills.

Now comes the task of decluttering and tidying the property to make it presentable. It's a huge job. Thankfully, the permaculture group, some of whom I've never even met before, come to my aid quite a few times over the next few months. My neighbours, Don and Kip, also do what they can.

My friend Tansy helps me interview real estate agents, and another friend advises on styling the house. So much to do. I borrow money from my friend Jo to pay for work to be done and upfront fees for the house sale. My friend Costa flies up to finish the wetlands area that has become a haven for my beautiful green tree frogs and a space of boundless peace and joy for me. Everyone agrees the property is too much for me to manage, and I need to take that stress off myself. I must admit, every time I drive into my property, all I can see is the huge amount work that needs to be done, but I don't know how I can make it all happen in time.

CHAPTER 22

Bright-Coloured Clothes

Each week for the last one or two years, I've gone to sound bowls therapy with David, and it's one of the most profound healing experiences I've ever had. I always come out feeling much better, my body resonating with sound. Tonight, David announces he's suspending these group sessions, and all future ones will be by invitation only. From this action, it seems to me he's saying he doesn't feel he's being respected for what he does.

There are only three of us in the room, including his best friend and my Lyme friend Brit. I always pay each week and make sure to tell him how much it helps us. It doesn't make any sense, and I'm deeply upset. How can he stop something that makes such a difference to our healing journey?

I can't sleep all night. In the morning I send a text thanking him for everything he's done for me over the years and say goodbye. He texts me the next day, and every day for quite some time, inviting me to his sound healings. I never reply. I don't understand what this is all about, but the damage is done. Brit also gets invited back but declines as well.

I go to a garden show at Gympie but don't last long, as I'm too tired. But apparently I didn't realize just how exhausted I was, as on my drive home, I'm not aware I'm going around those huge orange partitions that let you know the road is closed. I don't even have enough alertness to realise there aren't any other cars. All I can think about is getting home and getting into bed.

A policeman pulls me up and says, "Why are you driving on this road?" and I say, truthfully, "I'm going home. I'm so tired." Then my subconscious steps in, and I spit out a lie, which I'm not even aware of at the time. I say I live up the road (that only locals are allowed on), and the lovely policeman lets me drive on. I'm surprised he didn't give me a police escort to get me off the road. Thanks, Universe.

Everything's changing

I'm once again reminded of how much my life has changed, when the Queensland Garden Expo returns, I'm an emotional wreck. For approximately ten years, I've been part of this expo, from being on the organising committee and hands-on setting it up, to giving workshops and speaking at the event. It's also a fun opportunity to meet up with everyone from interstate.

Now I'm too sick to be a part of it, and it hurts me deeply. I can't stop crying. It once again makes me feel like I'm nothing. I can't do anything, and to be honest, most of the time when I'm out, I'm just faking that I'm okay to make others feel good.

Where has my life gone? When will I ever get better? What am I going to do with my life? I can't go anywhere, because I just keep crying. I feel like such a failure. My life is non-existent. I'm angry at the world. I hate having Lyme disease. I throw things at the wall, wishing I didn't have to do this alone.

I'm struggling with depression again. At least I'm more aware of it, but I know that if I'm still in the black hole after three days, I'm in deep trouble and need to seek professional help, or else it's too hard to climb out.

I make myself get out of bed, put on bright-coloured clothes, and go into town, where I at least have to see other people's faces, even if I don't know them. I try and snap myself out of this, but it's so hard. Being colourful helps, because people tend to smile at me, and colour has always made me feel happier. All of this, combined with leaving the house, helps me so much. But I keep my sunglasses on, just in case I'm crying behind them.

CHAPTER 23

That's What Friends Are For

More than ever, I need to increase my treatments to cope with the extra workload and pressure of selling the house This is what I'm doing to keep the pain at bay and to help me function:

- Going to the healing centre every week
- Massage
- Bioresonance
- Acupuncture
- PowerTube
- Brown's gas
- BioMat
- Infrared sauna
- Bicarb/magnesium detox baths
- Colonics
- Element 5 (for EMF)
- Physiotherapy
- Seeing a naturopath
- Mountains of supplements

- Bone broths
- Hertz music, meditation CDs at night

I'm still having so much trouble with radiation in my body. It doesn't make sense. I don't expose myself to it. I don't put my phone to my ear or on my body, I have EMF protection in the whole house, and when I go out, there are no towers anywhere nearby. My body is so sensitive to it, but my Lyme count has gone up, as have my heavy metals.

My body is really struggling, and I'm pushing it hard. There's so much pain going through me. I have constant headaches and feel overwhelmed, I'm still experiencing nausea in the morning, it's hard to breathe, and there's a weird pain above my right eye. There's also pain in my right ankle. I get little sleep at night when I sweat, and then I purge heat during day. But I have no choice. I have a house to sell, and I also have a deadline for *Organic Gardener* magazine. So I have to push through, even though I'm a fragile, exhausted, emotional bunny.

Two weeks before the house goes on the market, a photographer is coming to take images for the real estate agent, and I'm close to collapsing. My daughters have been home helping me, but there's still so much to do. I text Val, a permaculture friend, and ask her to come help. Unbeknownst to me, she sends a message to the whole permaculture network, asking members to "come and support Leonie to get her house on the market, so she can sell it and continue treatments to get well." Wow. I wondered why messages were coming through wishing me luck and apologising for not being able to make it.

Then all of these people turn up and work so hard with me. They leave before dark, and I keep going. Melika, thankfully, has made dinner, and when I go inside, she looks at me covered from head to toe in dust, all hot and sweaty, and says, "Have a shower first, Mum." Now the roles have reversed, and she's telling me what to do.

I lie in bed at night, my body screaming at me to stop. I'm not even sure how I'm still going. *I'm sorry, body, but I have to do this to make sure I get the maximum sale price for my home, so we can then get treatments to heal and be fully well, healthy, energetic, and happy again.*

It's interesting to note the friends who help. Besides the amazing Permaculture Noosa group, there are the ones who are either struggling with an illness themselves or caring for someone. The friends who are fully well are not the ones knocking on the door, sleeves rolled up, ready to go. I guess when you're not dealing with this kind of stress, you go on with your life.

CHAPTER 24

In My Element

October 2016

My house is officially on the market. An open house and garden tour have been organised, and I'm in my element, talking to a large group of people. ABC Radio is also here, and they interview me afterwards. I have such a lovely time sharing my love for my property, and I feel the old me come back as I speak to everyone. I'm feeling wonderful. It reminds me to *be generous, be positive, be happy, and be grateful*, which are all qualities I used to have.

My doctor isn't happy I won't take antibiotics, but I truly believe, especially after listening to the U.S.A. Lyme summit, that antibiotics for chronic Lyme is useless in curing the illness and will only destroy my gut. Antibiotics only help when you first get a bite. Yet still, my mother is on the same antibiotic mantra *every* time I phone her, and the conversation deteriorates from that point. She's completely unable to understand my choices in any way.

The constant tidying of the house, never my strong point, is gruelling. Having to pile extra things into my car (like the washing) at the last minute, with my dog sitting on top of it all, is getting so tiring. I need a break from all of this stress. I don't understand how people can waste so much time having a pristine house.

A plague of insects comes through my garden and completely destroys it. I can't believe the timing! It's a rare insect that has descended on the Coast. It's not just my garden that has been attacked, and there isn't a thing I can do about it.

CHAPTER 25

Plan B

18 November 2016

I sell my home, but the contract isn't yet unconditional. I don't get the price I want, but I can't cope with all of the accumulative stresses, and I need to move on. The bank evaluator for the buyer goes through the house, and she's like Sherlock Holmes on steroids, picky beyond being realistic, and suddenly both the real estate agent and I have this massive list of things to do/improve, before finance can be approved for the buyer. Thank goodness I keep a diary and can track who gave approval of wetlands, etc.

On 29 November, the contract goes unconditional. When I get the call, I scream like I've won Wimbledon and fall to the floor crying in relief. I don't think I realised how stressful all of this pressure has been, plus being in debt and not knowing my next step. Now I can go to my new doctor and try different treatments. I need to get well. There's no time to rest, though. It's a quick settlement, and I must pack up.

I phone Anne-Maree and thank her for always being there for me, plus, of course, the financial support and never questioning what I spent money on. I tell her that without her support, I wouldn't be above ground. I don't think she really understands how lost I would be without her emotional and financial support.

I have no plan B as to where I'll go once I move out of my home. I just don't have time to think about it. Thankfully, a horticultural friend, Tohm, comes to the rescue and says I can stay with him, until I find somewhere to live. I've also arranged to do some housesitting early next year.

The day before I leave, I'm sitting on my deck having a break, drinking a quiet herbal cuppa. The kookaburras are on the deck railing, which isn't unusual, except there are so many of them, but there's also king parrots, which have never before come onto the deck, and one is sitting on my rocking chair. Suddenly, with much emotion, I realise they know I'm leaving, and they've come to say goodbye to me. I've created a better home for them with more trees, scrubs, and natural food, and they're thanking me for it. I'm going to miss them all so much. I love everything I've created here on my organic permaculture property, all 1.5 acres of heaven backing onto a freshwater lagoon that has held me most mornings and sunsets. I'm not sure if my heart is bursting with love or breaking with sadness.

I'd been hoping to do some sort of goodbye ceremony to my land, the plants, and the animals on it, but I still have so much packing and cleaning to do, and I keep having to sleep to keep functioning. I fall into bed for the last time in my home. Potcy sleeps in my suitcase tonight. He knows something's going on.

The removalist arrives an hour early to take stuff to the storage container. I haven't finished packing or showering. It's all go, go, go. Melika arrives, and my friend Andrew, too, thank goodness.

I have everything labelled into three categories, so the removalist will know where to pack boxes in the container: P=permanent, which goes to the back, =R==rental, which goes in the middle, and A=easy access.

I then lead the removalist to the storage container, and while they're unloading, I race back home a half-hour drive away, as Andrew and Melika want some instructions on what to do next, plus the removal men have accidently taken the brooms, so I need to get back to sort out cleaning and final pack, before returning.

When I get back, the removalists are pleased to advise me that the container is fully packed. They open the door, and I see the wrong boxes at the front. Everything has been packed incorrectly. I just close my eyes and say to them, "Shut the door." I have no energy to deal with it.

Back home again, I send Melika and Andrew off. Potcy is going with Melika, but halfway up the drive, he turns and stares at me and will not move. The look on his face says, "Where are you going? Are you okay?" I can only urge him to get into Melika's car.

Once everyone has gone, I can finally say goodbye to the land and all of my animals that will be staying: The guinea pigs, chooks, frogs, birds, kangaroos, snakes, goannas, ducks, and swamp hens … as well as my food forest, vegetable garden, plants, wetlands, and all of the trees I've planted in memory of animals and friends. Then I bid farewell to the large rocks, boulders, and tree logs that were gifted to me for this landscape. So many plants from friends. I've put a lot of work and love into this land. My heart is going to break. I'm sobbing as I walk around the property slowly, apologising for leaving it and thanking it for nurturing and loving me.

"Oh, I'm going to miss you all so much," I say.

I hate that I have to sell my house, because of this goddam bastard of a disease. How could you be so cruel, Universe? I'm a good person. I was doing good things in the world … I love this land and did such wonderful things to improve it, to make it a better place for Mother Earth and all of her plants, birds, and animals. I hate you for doing this to me. This property has been such a healing space, and now you've taken it away from me. Why do good people get sick? Why don't the ones who don't give a shit about life and don't do anything, get sick? It's so unfair. Lyme, I hate what you've done to me. I have no life, and I've lost so much that is important to me…my work, my travel, my friends, my fun, my land, my animals, and my home.

When I finally get into my car and drive off, I can barely see, as I'm sobbing so much. I'm overwhelmed with grief. I'm a mess.

I have to stop the car and try to calm down before I get to Tohm's place. I've pre-warned him I might be upset, but I can't turn up looking a complete wreck. The grieving sobs keep pouring out, but I finally compose myself.

I'm so glad to arrive at his home, and he's there to hug me when I get out of the car, still crying. Thank goodness I'm staying with someone, as right now wouldn't be a good time to be alone in my grief. I have zero coping skills.

Tohm has set up the room beautifully. I have a much-needed shower while he cooks me dinner. I even have a beer. My grief is settling.

CHAPTER 26

Graduation Day

I have one day's rest before heading off to Fedora's graduation from Griffith University. I haven't driven to Brisbane for a couple of years, so just driving is going to be challenging enough. My body is running on zero everything. I'm completely shattered physically, emotionally, and mentally, with a nervous system that's fragile and jumpy. To top it off, I must play happy families with my ex-husband. You could say this situation is not what the psychologist ordered!

I find the hotel without getting too lost, book in, and have a quick lie down. I'm so tired and stressed from the car trip, but I made it.

When I wake up, I have to hit the ground running. I managed to pack the right dress, high shoes, and lipstick, so I'm off to a good start, but then I get a bit confused finding the graduation location. The girls are already in Brisbane having lunch with their dad.

I do find it, and the ceremony is good. I cheer loudly as my daughter is presented with her certificate, a double degree in business and psychology. I always joked that she did business to follow her father and psychology to work out her mother

After the family photos, the others decide we'll go to a bar. Oh, dear…sensory overload. Lots of people, and a loud band. They order food, but there isn't a thing I can eat that I won't react to. I feel so forgotten. They all know I have food restrictions. It's not like it's something new. My ex is bragging, as usual, about his latest purchases as my nervous system heads into overload, and I feel like I'm about to explode. Thankfully, for the third time in my life, I hear a loud voice in my head say, "Get up, and leave NOW."

I quickly say I have to go, kiss the girls goodbye, and walk outside, where I head for the river the opposite direction to my motel. I have no intention of going there yet. I need the solace of the water to calm me.

I get to the corner at the traffic lights and start crying. Five minutes later, I'm sitting on the grass by the river at Southbank, sobbing uncontrollably.

What has happened to my life! Why do I always look like the bad parent? I've lost my children. I've lost my land and my home. I've lost my health and vitality. I've lost my business and identity. I've lost friends. My family doesn't care about me, except for Anne-Maree. Why do I always end up looking like the worst person when there's a family event? Because I don't have money, all I can give is love, and apparently that isn't as good. It doesn't buy fun, adventure, travel, or useless things. I'm so sad. Why the fuck has this happened to me? Fuck you, Universe! When are you going to help me? I NEED YOUR HELP. I CAN'T KEEP DOING THIS. I'm not a fucking martyr.

I decide I'd better go to my motel, but I can't find it. I know it's close by, but every time I get to the bridge, I know I've gone too far. I take my phone out, but I can't understand how to read the map. It says I'm only minutes away, but I can't work out how to get there. I keep walking back to the river and start again. A guy walks past and says, "Good evening." Later, he passes me again and says, "God bless you." I want to reach out to him and say, "Please give me a hug." I don't, though. Instead, I continue to cry while walking back and forth, trying to find my motel. It takes hours, but eventually I can see the sign. When I get to my room, I know I can't stay there. I'm restless and hungry, so I put on some thongs and leave again. This time I record multiple landmarks, so I can find my way back. There's no way I'll miss the life-sized upside-down stone elephant, even though I can't work out the significance of it being outside of a library.

The crazy part is that I'm only a ten-minute walk from where I started. My brain just isn't functioning.

I get something to eat and sit on the grass, staring at the moon over the water … and cry some more. It's a full moon, and it's beautiful, but I'm swearing at it.

I've spent so much of my life being a great mum to my girls and giving them a loving experience, and yet none of that seems to be remembered. Their dad is the hero these days. My heart hurts so much. I wish they could understand just how hard this Lyme disease is, but I guess I did too good of a job playing it down for them.

As I wake up the next morning, I immediately start crying, so I go for a walk along the river and will myself to stop. I have an appointment with a new doctor in Brisbane today.

The doctor is straightforward about what he can do with treating me. I like what he has to say, as it's quite progressive, and he has the latest equipment from overseas. But he's also arrogant, with no shortage of ego. It doesn't matter, though. I want to end this Lyme story and get some fast results, and I have the money to do whatever treatment I want. I start the Hyperthermic Ozone and Carbonic Acid Transdermal Therapy (Hocatt™), as well as 10- Pass Ozone with him next month.

It's a long drive back home to Tohms, and I must remind myself to focus. When I get there, I'm so relieved that I can finally rest and restore my body and brain.

CHAPTER 27

Lesson Learned

January, 2017

I've stopped my Centrelink payments, because I realised that I'm never going to get well with the stress they constantly put me under. I'll finance myself with the money from the sale of my home. I can't believe how good this decision feels. I am free. No more shackles around my body. I no longer have to put up with the incompetence, rudeness, and lack of compassion/humanness from Centrelink/Human Resources. I'm feeling positive. I'm smiling. I feel like a bird that just found their wings.

I have my appointment with the Brisbane doctor's clinic. First, I receive the HocattTM hyperthermia with ozone and steam. It looks like some strange capsule with my head poking out the top. I'm in it for thirty minutes at 45–47 degrees Celsius (113 degrees Fahrenheit). The last eight minutes, I feel a bit dizzy.

I dry off, dress, and go into another room, where I sit in a comfy chair and have a needle inserted into my arm for the 10-Pass Ozone. It takes sixty–ninety minutes. I don't feel anything and just listen to a podcast. Afterwards, the nurse asks what IV supplements I want. I ask, "What does the doctor recommend?" and she says, "People usually have magnesium and vitamins B & C." She made figuring out which IV supplements I should have sound like choosing lollies at a shop. I had the ones she suggested. Obviously, they cost a lot more than lollies.

Side-effects were expected. I have daily massive headaches and feel sick for days as I struggle with the summer heat. For the next two weeks I'm house sitting in Brisbane. The house is filthy, and I have to spend my precious energy cleaning it. I even wash the kitchen floor with boiling water to sterilise it. Thankfully, my bedroom is clean.

At my appointment for my second dose of hyperthermia and 10-Pass Ozone, I really struggle with the hyperthermia and ask for it to be turned off five minutes before the end, as I feel like I'm going to be sick, and I'm dizzy. The nurse tries to talk me into staying longer, but I don't give up easily and am always aware when I've pushed my body. I know I'm at breaking point.

She opens the door, and I nearly fall out. I'm so weak and sick, I sit there with my head in my hands. Eventually, I dress and go to the IV room for 10-pass and IV supplements.

All week, I feel soooo sick, and it's hard to breathe. I walk around holding my liver, and I'm still not coping well with the current heatwave. My perception of where I am has completely gone, and I'm scared to walk beyond the end of the road in case I can't remember how to get back to my house.

I keep taking notes about everything, as my memory is non-existent. I don't know what's happening, and it's scary.

Eventually, I think of a natural practitioner I can go to. They're bio-resonance people I've been to before and liked.

When I walk in, the practitioner takes one look at me and tells me to sit. "Leonie," she says, "your reactions are so slow. Your energy is at a dangerously low level, and nothing will be getting through to your brain. You should not be driving! The state of your health at present is diabolical." And my classic response to this is, "I'm fine driving!! It's walking that's a problem. I don't know where I am." Wow! That's a rude awakening. My car's GPS is making me feel safe and competent. Scary.

All she can do to help me is try to give my body some energy, and it can't cope with anything more than that. She won't even put me on the bio-resonance machine. I'm also forever grateful that she warns me about my current Brisbane doctor giving me the treatments. She says, "He's renowned for pushing patients to the edge. Be very careful, Leonie."

I thankfully take her warning and stop further hyperthermia but keep emailing the doctor to let him know how sick I am and that I can't move off the couch due to my nausea, headaches, exhaustion, and having no energy. He doesn't respond. This is when I need a partner to take over and deal with the problem.

I feel like shit. I lie on the couch moaning, still holding onto my stomach and liver, due to internal pain. I'm pale, and I can't stop sweating. Everything hurts, and I can't think. I hate the bright glow of the sun and the lights in the room at night, as well as the noises of the neighbourhood. I'm also emotional, so I decide to listen to some meditations that will keep me calm and focussed beyond my body.

I've been posting on Facebook about what's been going on, and two friends offer to collect me and bring me back home again, which is a two-hour drive away. One of them is a friend with Lyme, and the other has cancer. Once again, I'm reminded that it's the friends experiencing illness who are the first ones coming to my aid.

I let them know I'll drive back, because otherwise I'll have to make another trip to collect my car. Potcy dog came with me on this house sit, so I have him to keep me company. I'm sick, sad, crying, and missing my old home. I have one more 10-pass Ozone treatment coming up, and eight IVs of Phosphatidylcholine to go, but I'm not getting anywhere near the Brisbane doctor again.

CHAPTER 28

Three Positive Things

When I see my home doctor and acupuncturist, both are really upset about my appalling state of health "Your organs have been cooked!!! Even if the Brisbane doctor did kill off the Lyme, it would come back, as your whole immune system has been wiped out."

All of my practitioners are kind to me over the next few months as I slowly rebuild my immunity and strength. Once I feel better, I do some more research, and apparently no hyperthermia treatment place goes over forty-two degrees! No wonder I struggled with it. Probably lucky I had the 10-Pass Ozone and IVs to help keep my body going.

If I were a little child again, I would probably say to my mother, "Mummy I'm not going to the doctor anymore. They make me sick and hurt me.'

I'm not having a good run with doctors this year, so once again I decide to take control and run with the latest book/podcast I've been following from a U.S. doctor. He suggests doing a strict detox diet for twenty-eight days. I figure it can't hurt. In my effort to try and stay positive, even with setbacks in my progress, I convince myself that there are still more lessons for me to learn, more knowledge to gather, and more people to meet. But this hope can run thin … wafer thin! What I need is a crystal ball.

I'm seeing another psychologist, but honestly, I'm not there to tell them all of the latest treatments for Lyme when they're fascinated by my journey, especially when I'm paying. I know what I'm doing for Lyme, and that I have the physical symptoms under control. It's all the trash in my head I need to get rid of and to acquire some coping mechanisms.

I'm much better off seeing a kinesiologist, who can tap into me straight away and clear up my crap negative core beliefs.

I'm house sitting at various locations. I couldn't stay with Tohm forever, although his friendship, hospitality and generosity were enormously appreciated and needed. At some housesits I'm allowed to bring Potcy, but otherwise, he goes to my daughter Fedora's in Brisbane. I like being in new towns and locations and exploring them, but being in different homes is wearing thin. Each time I leave, I have to do a huge clean, as I always leave the house tidier than when I arrived. It takes a huge amount of strength out of me. Friends are kind in offering a room for me when I'm in-between house sits, especially my permaculture friend Penny and her hubby Lindsay, as well as Noely and Stephen.

I keep two journals that are essential for my sanity. There's my everyday journal that I speak to like a friend. It holds no judgement, doesn't comment, and never interrupts. This is my diary where I write all of my fears, joys, hurts, pains, anger, and things I love, too. My other journal, *What are three positive things in my day?*, sits by my bedside. No matter how bad my day has been, I'll always find three positive things, even if it's *I'm grateful for my legs and being able to walk. I have a bed; a roof over my head, and a toilet.* Honestly sometimes I stretch to come up with positives, but really, there are plenty. I just need to think differently.

I also have a diary that's more like an exercise book that I keep outside of my bedroom. Before going to bed. I write in it everything that I'm upset or worried about and ask the Universe to take care of it while I'm sleeping/resting. This is to elevate my mind to stop it from spinning all night with problems.

By March, I've had enough of house sitting and need to be still. I'm renting the bottom level of a friend's three-storey beachside apartment across from my favourite beach, Point Arkwright, on Queensland's Sunshine Coast. It has lots of great big rocks I can sit on and watch the water beneath.

Each day, I head to the beach in the early morning and again in the evening, where I lap up the sun in my bikinis and practise relaxing. I'm not used to having nothing to do. I have no animals or gardens to look after or work to run off to. It takes a few weeks to be peaceful and relax.

I still sleep most days and have lots of appointments. My lungs are a worry, and when I get tired, my breath gets hot and thick, but it settles once I've slept. And though breathing can be difficult, especially when I lie down, sometimes I find the sound of my laboured breath soothing in a weird way, and I fall asleep. It's like it's some crazy new meditation technique: focus on your breathless breath!

My nervous system is painful, especially when I lie down, and often I don't like to recline, knowing it means pain throughout my body. Also, there's the heat purge just before I fall asleep, which wakes me up completely as I roll around the mattress looking for cold spots. And then there's the brain fog. I'm sure there's a memory vault inside my head; I just need to find the key!

I feel so lonely. I'm my only cheer squad, and sometimes I wonder why I'm doing so much to try and get well. What's the purpose?

But I continue on trying to rebuild my tired body and spirit. Though I'm too worn-out to cook, I'm eating one or two meals, plus juices, from the local organic vegetarian café.

I've also found a local doctor here to give me the last few IVs. As the nurse is putting the needle in, she misses my vein, and I scream in pain. She takes it out and gets the doctor, who's nurturing and soothing. He reinserts the needles elsewhere, and from then on, I never let the nurse near me.

I'm starting to go out in public more, but to places where people are unlikely to recognise me. I don't want to wear the Lyme label, and if I'm around people who don't know me, I can pretend I'm well and still working in organic gardening. I also go to talks at the local libraries, which helps my brain re-engage.

With my chemical sensitivity, I have to make sure I don't sit anywhere near a smoker, due to the smell lingering on their clothing, anyone who wears perfume, uses spray deodorants, or wears clothes washed in fragrant laundry detergents.

My new local friend, Tansy Grant, has been good to me over the months and is always so positive and a breath of fresh air. She's taken over caring for Potcy. Sometimes my ex picks up the dog for a few days, and one time when I come to collect him, I notice he has one eye shut. Of course, the ex is oblivious to the dog's discomfort.

It turns out he has an eye infection, which means weeks of collecting the dog from Tansy and taking him to the vet. I'm twenty-five minutes from Tansy, and then then it's another fifteen minutes in the opposite direction to the vet's. By the time I get done with all of that driving, I can barely move.

CHAPTER 29

I'm Allowed

I book a free one-day personal development course with Authentic Education in Brisbane and a room for two nights at the hotel where the event is being held, so I can have all of my home-cooked food in my room and sneak back there for a quick rest. I'm hoping I can manage being at this course. The main reason I'm going is that I need to have some focus in my life going forward.

Before I leave for Brisbane, I get a call from another friend who'd been to visit Potcy while Tansy is away, and she says he seems worse. I close my eyes and take a deep breath. I can't believe this is happening. My relaxing, stress-free day suddenly does a backflip. Now I'm taking a forty-minute drive to the vet and back. By this stage, I need to sleep. Once I've rested, I drive ninety minutes to Brisbane, and I need another nap. Then I get a chance, just before sunset, to have a quiet walk along the river and through the gardens at Southbank.

I'm finally at the one-day course. It's exciting to be amongst non-Lyme people where no one knows my story, and I can pretend to be normal. I must be driving the presenter, Benjamin Harvey, crazy, as I keep playing with my eyes trying to get them to stay open. My head droops forward occasionally as I nod off, and I'm constantly restless in my seat. The day is much harder for me than I'd imagined.

But the two words repeated by Ben that resonate with me are, I'M ALLOWED! For years, no one has told me that. All I've heard constantly is, "Leonie, don't do this," and "Don't do that," and "No, you can't." Even though it isn't directly aimed at me, and is a marketing tool, it's totally winning me over. It reminds me that I have no one controlling me. I'm in charge of my new life and my destiny! No one can stop me. I need something to look forward to, but not to be doing it all on my own again, which I did with my edible school gardens program.

So, you guessed it, I buy some courses from them. But I'm so tired, so utterly fatigued and actually feeling sick by the end of the day, I can't even fill out the form, and one of the staff has to do it for me…not that they mind, of course. Mentally, I'm so happy and excited, but physically, my body is giving me a beating. I really hate the pain that shoots throughout my nervous system in protest. Happy brain, unhappy body.

Potcy is back at the vet again. At one stage, the vet explains he needs an eye operation and will be kept overnight, so he needs to be cuddled and cared for. I look at the vet, completely drained of energy, and say, "Who looks after me?" The vet gives me a strange look, but the thought of renting a kennel for the night and having someone nurture ME, sounds like heaven.

Potcy is the family's dog, and the girls and the ex are all worried about him, so I give them updates each time I see the vet. Tansy helps take some of the driving pressure off me, as she can see I have no energy. The operation goes well.

I get a couple of abusive texts from the ex, and when I notice the date on my phone, I have to laugh. It's six years ago today since

I left him, and these texts confirm that I did the right thing. I'm sad that he treats me with no respect and has no compassion, even though I'm the mother of his children. I seem to have become the punching bag during Potcy's prolonged eye problems.

The vet and I decide Potcy shouldn't to be moved from Tansy's home, as it's too distressing for him not knowing where he is. Both eyes have been operated on, and he can't see.

Fedora arrives the next weekend, and against my instructions, she collects Potcy from Tansy's house and takes him for the weekend. I'm totally shattered, emotionally and physically. I don't have a gram of energy left in my body to deal with extra vet visits, not to mention the money it's costing me.

I can only sink to the floor and cry. I'm so tired and can't believe more unnecessary layers are being added. I go to the beach across the road to sit on my favourite rock, where I cry and cry and cry all day. I'm numb. No one cares about the toll this has taken on me. I can't do this anymore. And when I go to bed, I don't sleep…again.

It's Easter Sunday, and Fedora and her boyfriend Brock are here for lunch. I confront Fedora about taking Potcy, but she's definite about her right to collect her dog. I serve lunch. Everything comes out of a plastic bag, which is so against my healthy beliefs/standards. I just drop the contents onto the plates. I don't give a shit about preparing food or eating it. My nervous system is shot.

I hold back the tears until they leave. My heart is breaking. No one is supporting me, or even respecting me. I'm not in a good space.

That night, at one a.m., I get ready to phone the helpline of Beyond Blue (or maybe Black Dog, I can't remember which one).

It's a support service for anxiety, depression, and suicide. I check their website for a phone number, but before I dial, I'm distracted by a YouTube video, which I click onto. It tells me to have a support team of friends to call on … which just sets me off. My irrational mind goes into overdrive, and I yell at the screen, "No one will be awake at one a.m.! My support team is tired. They've been looking after me for four years already!" I don't make the phone call. I'm now angry and can't see how they could understand. I give up.

I decide to at least be productive and write my eulogy. I enjoy thinking of the people who do love me, and I give a heartfelt thanks and tears for their love and friendship. I'll miss them. I'm ready to say goodbye to the world. I can't see me ever being well enough to enjoy life again. There isn't a thing to look forward to. I'm never going to get well. I just need to wait another two days for those damn tourists to leave after Easter, so I can go down to my favourite beach across the road and do a one-way swim at night when no one's around. I've had enough. I can't do this anymore. I'm okay with my decision. I'm tired of fighting, and I'm not scared of dying.

The next day, I get an email from a guy named Frank, who I met years ago at a Toowoomba gardening expo I was speaking at. He asks me, *Are you okay? Are you ready to work again?* I reply, *I'm still sick and not able to work*. He writes back, *I'm here if you need someone to talk to, and I'm good at jokes*. I don't want to speak to anyone, but we continue emailing that afternoon. It was as if he knew I needed help that day, and this was enough to snap me out of my hypnotic state of hopelessness.

I don't do my one-way swim.

CHAPTER 30

Making A Difference

I spend the next few weeks having lots of appointments to boost my low self-esteem, depression, grief, and tired body. I'm in a desperate state of nothingness.

However, while sitting on my favourite rocks on the beach at Point Arkwright contemplating my world, through these moments of silence, I see this tiny bright light at the end of my long, dark tunnel, and a little voice reminds me, "'You have your new course in Sydney coming up. You're creating a new life and making a difference!" Yes! Thank goodness I have something to look forward to. Remembering the course and the new life purpose it can bring me, has given me a tiny little spark of future belonging. Lyme is such a journey.

One day, when the ex was collecting Potcy from Tansy for a visit, Tansy's husband blasted him and told him to take responsibility for the dog, meaning to take him permanently. Although I miss my beautiful, healing dog, it's become too stressful and exhausting for me, and it's not fair on Tansy trying to care for a dog that isn't well and not her responsibility. I need time to heal myself.

In May 2017, I feel strong enough to drive to Toowoomba, three hours away, to visit my friends, Bevan and Maureen. I stay there for a couple of days, and we go to local farms and gardens. I thoroughly enjoy my time. It's great to be welcomed into their home and have meals cooked for me.

Many of my practitioners and healers are now my friends. It's easy to see why I became close to them, as they're the few people who truly understand the pain, grief, and uncertainty of my illness.

I love going to my chemist, LiveLife Pharmacy in Noosa, run by naturopaths. David, Rochelle, Colleen, and Nat have been a lifeline to me on many occasions. They know me so well. I can never pretend I'm fine, as they see right through me. If I walk in feeling sad, they know just how to cheer me up, until I'm belly laughing with their jokes, stories, and songs. I leave feeling absolutely wonderful, smiling and laughing as I drive home. I think about how this is the old me. It's what I used to do all the time: laugh, joke, smile, and radiate joy. What happened to the old Leonie?

When I get home, I take a big piece of paper and write *WHO IS LEONIE? WHERE HAS SHE GONE?* Then I write in different coloured texts all of my good qualities that I've forgotten: *joyful, laughs, jokes, sings, dances, is positive, energetic, compassionate, helpful, fun, loving, generous, loyal, friendly, inspirational, radiant, colourful, intelligent, and is a good speaker and gardener.*

I put that on the wall where I'll see it each day, so I can remember who I am and practise being me again. It's a powerful moment.

CHAPTER 31

I Have The Power

Against all logic, common sense, and sanity, I'm risking flying to Sydney for my new courses. I've done a lot of preparation for this journey to make sure I'm strong enough and protected from EMF, radiation, and chemicals, so I don't end up in hospital again.

Some of the processes include:

- not flying between eight a.m. and five p.m.
- sitting at the back of the plane on an aisle seat, farthest away from the cockpit and windows
- being well rested and hydrated
- eating healthy food
- taking a whole range of different supplements before and after the flight.

I also have a special blanket I wrap around me that protects me from EMF. Apparently, there's a cap to protect your brain while flying, but I draw the line at the blanket. I already look strange enough.

In order to build my immunity and protect my brain and body, I set up a schedule of what I need to do before, during, and after the flight. Again, this is not medical advice.

Start taking three weeks before flying	Astaxanthin and other powerful antioxidants Matcha green tea powder probiotics
Eat	Organic almonds, berries, broccoli, cabbage, cauliflower, citrus, dark chocolate, flax seeds (food for lungs, too), dark green leaves, mustard, rosemary, turmeric, and walnuts. Fermented food, chlorophyll-rich foods, seaweed, kelp, spirulina, and chlorella, iodine.
Supplements	SAMe between meals, Vitamins A, C & E, Zinc, Selenium, Liquorice, Indian gooseberry, NAC, Omega 3, Quercetin, and resveratrol.
Protection on the plane	Don't touch mouth, nose, or eyes. Spray Thieves in mouth and around seat.
After landing	Earthing on grass, beach, or forest.
Bath	Epsom and baking soda for twenty to thirty minutes.
Additional	IR sauna to release the toxins from flying. Zeolite/bentonite clay (detoxing) each day. Continue minerals as above. Dandelion, peppermint, chrysanthemum to detox.

I'm the last person to get on the plane. Thankfully, no one is in the seat next to me, and the other person by the window is a friendly lady.

I'm struggling to get the special EMF protection blanket around me, which honestly is like wrapping myself in cardboard. I've practised doing this at home, but there isn't much space in the plane. The lovely lady helps me, and I'm so embarrassed, I want to cry, but I don't.

The lady and I have an in-depth conversation about health, as she, too, is having her own challenges. What I thought would be a difficult time turned out to be a quick and relaxing flight with insightful conversation.

I arrive at the course a day early, so I can familiarise myself with where everything is and to cook my food. There are too many noises and smells, a lot of people smoking outside buildings, and the busyness of Sydney is slightly overwhelming for me.

The course has about 150 participants and goes for eight hours a day for six days, with homework each night. It's full-on, and I'm not coping well, often crying several times a day due to being depleted.

By lunchtime on day three, I'm an emotional mess. I'm like a two-year-old who's over-tired and just cries. Ben asks me what's going on, and I finally stop crying enough to be able to say, "I'm sooo tired! I have Lyme disease. I thought I could do this, but I can't."

The next words that Ben says are so insightful, it energizes me straight away. He says, "Leonie, there are lots of people out there who claim to be experts but have never actually experienced the problem, so imagine the power you could have by actually sharing your experience and knowing firsthand how your life looks and the way to get well from information not found in textbooks."

Well, that certainly dries up my eyes and puffs out my chest. Not only *can* I do this, I *need* to do this, so I can go out and help others. Thank you, Ben!

I soon realise it's hard to keep to my schedule, as the timing of our breaks doesn't match when I need to eat food. So much new information is coming into my brain, and being around new people and experiences is consuming huge amounts of energy, that I need to replenish often. I need full meals and both first and second breaks to keep me going.

One day, as we all pile into the lift to go home, people ask me if I'm coming out to dinner with the group. I just stare at them and calmly tell them I can't, almost in fear thinking I must find more energy to keep going. I would love to be social, but going out to dinner is definitely not in the cards if I want to keep functioning.

I don't last the whole course. I give up on day five, as I just can't manage any more. But that's okay. I love what I've achieved, especially being around new people and hearing about their futures.

One of the reasons I booked with this training company was that I can come back and redo the course anytime within three years, which means I can really nail it next time. Even though I'm tired, and it will take some weeks to recover, mentally, it's done so much for my future belonging and wellbeing. To actually believe that there's a new future out there for me, where I can help people, so they don't have to go through what I have. I can teach them the true path to wellness. It's lovely to have my confidence boosted and feel that I have a team around me to support me through my new journey.

CHAPTER 32

A Good Detox

My weeks are full of appointments in my quest to become well, along with lots of sleeping. My regular health practitioners and loyal supporters are my doctors, naturopath, bioresonance machine, Chinese medicine, acupuncture, and healing group each Monday. Of course, there's also a list a mile long of other treatments:

- hyperbaric oxygen therapy (HBOT)
- lymphatic massage
- colonics
- reiki
- pulsed electromagnetic field (PEMF) therapy
- Biomat™ (infrared rays and negative ions) with IR sauna
- PowerTube
- lymphasizer trampoline
- coffee enemas
- Brown's gas

In addition, Keryn, a healer from Perth, remotely infuses energy into my drinking water for the day. I also do toning (music and voice), and have the occasional tuning forks. As a Lyme patient, I'll try anything to increase the building blocks of health.

The most important element for anyone who's struggling with a chronic illness, is having the support of friends ... and they may not be the ones you would expect. It will hurt deeply that many of them will walk away from you in your time of need, but this opens the space for new people to come into your life who are there to heal and support you fully. It can be a good detox of friends and relatives, which allows you to bring in healthier, more loving people.

CHAPTER 33

Happy Adrenals

For the first time in years, I'll be back speaking at the 2017 Queensland Garden Expo. This used to be my biggest event for the year, and I'm determined to be well enough to not only do a fabulous talk, but also the best one ever. I need to be back on stage again to see if I can still do it and attract a crowd.

Over the years, some fellow horticulturalists have said to me, "You'll never get back speaking now. You've been out of it too long." I'm here to prove them wrong. For the next few months, and in the lead-up to the garden expo, I have a strong focus and purpose, making it so much easier to be strict with my health routines and food...not that I eat any junk food... and making sure I'm balanced between excitement and rest, rest, rest.

July 2017 Queensland Garden Expo

I'm radiating with excitement, which is not exactly what the adrenals ordered, and positive energy. This is such an important milestone in my journey, and I'm not going to stuff up. I need to be good. I'm speaking after lunch and planned not to arrive until midday, but I'm excited and want to see everyone, so I leave mid-morning. However, when I get halfway through the thirty-minute drive, I realise I'm not going to make it if I don't stop. My adrenals aren't happy with me. I stop by a river and meditate to calm my nerves and excitement. I must conserve energy, so I eat some of the food I've packed and have a rest before driving the rest of the way to the expo.

When I arrive, I go to the VIP tent to put my food in the fridge. I get such a warm welcome from EVERYONE. Lots of hugs and kisses, and everyone can't help but notice my positive energy. My talk is really good. I feel confident and have no nerves. Most of the marquee is full. I stumble a bit when I see two senior horticultural people in the audience, but I just say to everyone, "Why is it you get more nervous when your friends are in the audience?" and get back on track.

Horticulture friends have turned up to support me, which is huge, and I'm grateful to them. I sell heaps of my book *Eat Your Garden: Organic Gardening for Home and School,* and sign most of them. It always amuses me that people want me to sign books.

That night, at a horticulture dinner, when anyone asks me how it went, I say, "I was great!" I'm so proud of myself. It's a huge milestone. Few people really understand what an achievement today's talk was. It was so important for my sense of purpose, belonging, and mental health.

Not surprisingly, I don't sleep much, as my body hits back with pain surging through my nervous system, and my everything aches when I lie down. But my mental health just had a massive boost of feeling of value to the world.

The next day at the expo, I'm not quite so energetic, but I still love being around everyone. My body is screaming at me to go home and rest, but this event is like a reunion for me, catching up with gardening friends from all over Australia, so I push myself through it, knowing I'm going to pay for it in the following days/weeks.

And boy was I right. For the next two weeks, I barely sleep, even though I'm spent, but I have so much shooting pain going through me. I'm honouring what my body needs after I pushed it, so now I'm just resting most of the day, every day. But even through it all, I'm so happy to have made this huge step forward. I will be quiet for the rest of the year, so I can get through the next stage of my health.

I have a new Lyme-literate doctor, and though he isn't allowed to say he treats patients for Lyme illness, I'm keen to progress forward with him. I'm also taking bucketloads of supplements.

Unfortunately, where I'm renting isn't good for resting. It's too hot in my room, too small, and too noisy. For now, I'll make the most of the beach across the road. I love going there, and the ocean is so healing.

CHAPTER 34

Fix Me!

August/September 2017

I'm pissed off with life. My health is getting worse, but thank God for my wonderful naturopath/bioresonance man, Mark, who listens to me and finds answers. Mark is so patient with me, as I often take out my frustration on him (sorry, Mark). For the last three months, my bowels have got worse and worse, with up to eight-plus bowel movements a day, every day. I don't want to leave the house, because I only get a second's warning before my bowels explode. No one knows what's causing it. I don't even want to eat. There seems no point. I'm losing weight, and I'm so tired. I went on my doctor's 'emergency' waiting list to see him, but still no phone call. He's always hard to get an appointment with.

I send an SOS that reads, *MARK, YOU HAVE TO FIX ME!!!!!* He orders special syrups from the U.S.A., and tablets from somewhere else, but he still couldn't work out why it was happening.

Meanwhile, Rasunah has me speak to a bowel guy in Sydney, and he's saying, "You need to do this and that etc., etc.," and I say, "I already do all of that!" Then he goes, "Really?". But three days after I receive the drops from Mark, I go back to three normal craps just like that! There's much 'relief' for everyone concerned. I'm so grateful to Mark for finding a solution. Those potions worked.

When I finally get to see the doctor, I have a list of tests I want done to figure out what's going on, which includes the kidneys, liver, homocysteine, and methylation. Naturopath Mark is so good and checks on me all the time. I'm grateful for his support and that he doesn't get cross with me when I yell at him in frustration to fix me.

My immunity is shot, and so is my absorption. I just keep taking all of the stuff the bioresonance machine says I need and hope my cells grab some of it on the way through. It's bloody expensive. The number of tablets and potions I take every single day is crazy. My mountain of supplements makes the Egyptian pyramids look insignificant. But I want to keep improving, so I continue and am grateful I have the funds from selling my home to support it.

I was meant to go camping with a healing friend. We were going to drive to Alice Springs and spend some time with the indigenous people, as I have a strong belief that our Aboriginals know the solution for Lyme. And I was going to catch up with my good friend Fiona, as well. But everything went wrong for him, so he cancelled. This turned out to be lucky, because even though I desperately wanted to go camping, I don't know how I thought I was going to manage with the way my body is currently functioning. It hasn't been a fun time, and it doesn't help that I'm restless.

I'm moving around a bit, trying to escape the renovations/facelift at the apartment block where I'm renting. There's noise, more noise, toxic crap, and more noise. I don't know what's happening with my life and just need to get away from everyone and everything, but especially from my rigorous routine. To be honest, I need someone to look after me. My diet is so restrictive that I'm getting to the stage where I'm too tired to work out what I can eat, and I just have grain-free toast. Tansy has recommended the Krishna village near Tyalgum in New South Wales as a retreat. It sounds fabulous, and I book it. I pack my car with my special Biomat that I sleep on, my pills, and potions. Where I'm going, there will be no coffee enemas, colonics, appointments, or noise.

I absolutely *love* the place. It's surrounded by hills, a flowing river, cows, and healthy, happy people. It takes me a couple of days to work out how to do nothing, and then I get quite good at it! I'm so nurtured. All meals are provided, and they're healthy and abundant. Before we eat, there's singing of gratitude for this food, and it's so special and uplifting. Everyone is friendly, and I enjoy the youthful energy of the people staying here.

After spending only six days in this place, I'm not ready to go home. There's a tearful goodbye and a promise to be back (for *my* sanity, not theirs). It was soooo good for me to be NURTURED. The joyfulness of the place and the singing of gratitude, not to mention having someone cook for me three times a day while seated cross-legged on the floor, and having a fascinating assortment of people to get to know, reinvigorated me. I try to bring that same joyfulness into my mealtimes at home, but singing alone isn't the same. Later, I find out they were discreetly checking on me, as they could see I wasn't well.

I travel to my friend Tohm's again for house sitting, and we catch up before he leaves. He has many fun, interesting stories to share and always makes me laugh. I love the peacefulness and beauty of his property, and I get to cook in a complete kitchen, walk on lush grass, and talk to chickens. The house sit goes too quickly.

When I return to my apartment after the peacefulness of the country, I realise I have to leave ASAP. This place has served its purpose, but it's time to be on my way. The Universe is pushing me as well. I just wish it would show me the crystal ball and let me know what the f*$%#* I'm meant to be doing with my life.

I'm grateful to have been opposite the beach, which has been so healing. The waves have collected my tears, allowed me to yell abuse and anger at the Universe, and beg it to help me. I've had plenty of joyful times of singing, dancing, absorbing the sun's positive rays, and rejoicing in how wonderful the world is. I've been so lucky to feel the sand between my toes and the sun and sea breeze on my skin as I sit on those solid rocks and watch the moving waves, always setting their own rhythm.

I feel my strength returning.

CHAPTER 35

Road Trip

My next house sit isn't for another three months, and my only commitment is to write for *Organic Gardener* magazine, which I can do from anywhere. I decide to go on a road trip to Victoria, my home state. My younger daughter, Melika, has been at Melbourne University for two years, and it hurts that I haven't been able to visit her. If I'm strict with myself and drive a maximum of three-hundred kms a day, take as long as I like, never drive at night, stop every three or four days, and listen to my body whenever it's had enough, I should be able to do it. I'll also need to stay in cabins or Airbnb's, as I need a kitchen to cook food.

I leave a few weeks later. I'm nervous, as I'm deliberately stepping back from the security blanket of ALL of my supportive naturopaths, doctors, healers, etc. Many have said I can phone them, but it's not the same as face to face, especially if I get really sick. I've ordered seven weeks of supplements/medication to carry with me in two big eskies in the car. You can imagine how big my Visa card bill is after those investments. I pack minimal clothes, non-perishable foods, my mineralised water, some treatment equipment, my Biomat, PowerTube and Brown's gas, as well as books and writing paper. My car is completely full.

I knew I would be exhausted before I even started the trip, so I booked the Krishna retreat again for a few days of love, gratitude, and rest upon my return.

The road trip is a book in itself. I drive along, looking at everything as if it's new and absolutely beautiful, because I never thought I would ever, ever, ever get to experience going on a holiday again or enjoy being in nature for extended periods. And I definitely could not have imagined I would be brave enough to drive myself all that way.

I'm in love with this panoramic country of Australia, which I call home. I stop constantly to take photos, hug an old tree, sit quietly by a waterway, eat lunch, stretch, close my eyes, and be silent. Wow! This is a truly amazing experience. I feel as if I've been given another chance at life. Like I've been born again into joy and beauty.

I stay off the main highways and have no plans except to be in Melbourne to see my daughter in three weeks. I never know where I'm going until the night before. I just point my finger south on the map and head in that direction without any researching. This is an adventure; I don't care which way I go. I love everything I see and being by myself.

I seem to fall upon festivals and great places to stay, although at one Airbnb, when I go canoeing on a river downstream, I struggle to paddle back. Thankfully, I manage to avoid a panic attack with lots of self-talk about how I'm safe and strong. This scare was a reminder that I'm not as fit as I was years ago.

My first stop on the Victorian/New South Wales border is to see my Aunty Valda and my cousins. When I arrive, I'm the happiest and healthiest I've felt for years. Aunty Val and I talk and laugh all afternoon. She's always stayed in touch with me, and I can sense her relief when she sees me well and happy. We get together again the next day, and I tell her I'll be back in three weeks when I'm on my way home. Then I visit my Aunty Trish, who was married to my late Uncle Digger. We used to spend every holiday at their home as kids, which backs onto the Murray River, so we spent a lot of time in the water. I created so many joyful memories.

At last I reach Melbourne, where I'll finally see Melika and where she lives and studies. We meet in the city and join in with a pro-gay/lesbian rally in support of the upcoming vote to legalise gay marriage in Australia. We go to parks and cafes, where I try to find food I can eat. It's so great to finally be here, but I'm tired and have to push my body.

From Melbourne, I go to my family hometown of Bendigo for the week, but unfortunately, my ol' friends and family seem to be too busy with their routines. I catch up with my friends' parents, now all in their eighties and nineties, as is my mum, and realise as I say goodbye to them that this will possibly be the last time I'll see some of them. I feel a little sad but am so grateful I decided to come back home to visit. They all played such a big role in my upbringing.

I'm enormously disappointed with everyone else. I thought that since I was sick when I was here a few years ago, they might be excited that I'm now so much better and celebrate with me over a mineral water.

After spending a lot of time doing nothing in Bendigo, I drive to my good friend Jo in Ballarat, who spoils me, and we visit lots of amasing gardens. Over the next couple of weeks, I stay with other friends around Victoria, Gavin, Kim, Cathy, and Merran. They also spoil me rotten and nurture me, even sending me off to bed for an afternoon nap when they see I'm tired. I feel so loved and cherished. I forgot how close I was to so many of these old friends and reflect that we all have our own journeys to deal with. I wish I could stay here for months to spend quality time with everyone.

I text my cousins to check if it's okay to stay with them on my return trip to Yarrawonga and catch up. They reply that my Aunty Val's health has declined dramatically and is on her deathbed. I arrive and get to spend twenty-four hours with her and all of her extended family, before she dies. WOW. What a special moment. I've never been around death before and have definitely been afraid of it, but it was one of the most beautiful experiences, with her bedside full of the people who treasured her most and shared that adoration with her. Aunty Val was definitely a much-loved woman.

The next day, I pack up and continue on. I know I'll be tired, because it's been such an emotional couple of days, plus being busy helping with the family cooking, etc. Half an hour after leaving, I can barely keep my eyes open, and I'm in so much pain. I stop at a tiny caravan park and get a cabin with a spa as a special treat.

I have trouble being upright, with shooting pain pumping through my nervous system. I feel so sick, and every part of my body is screaming. I'm actually scared I've pushed myself too hard this time. All day, I focus on restoring my body and feel thankful I'm travelling with lots of different health equipment.

The next day, I almost crawl to reception to book another night. I'm not good. But the following day, I'm feeling better. I know I've done lots of damage, but I don't regret my time with my aunty and my cousins.

I arrive in the Blue Mountains, my favourite place in Australia, and stay in the most perfect Airbnb with a woman with similar values. I love being in the mountains, with the rocks, the walks, the water, the clouds, the silence, and the cool. Every day I go walking in perfect peace and quiet, undisturbed by anyone else. It's restorative for the mind, body, and soul.

I leave this place so at peace, but then comes days of massive stress and getting close to a meltdown due to the traffic, trucks, getting lost, not being able to find my accommodation, and my car breaking down. What happened to people stopping to help when they see a woman with a broken car? I can't deal with stress, and I hate busy highways.

I'm in some country town where I book a room, as I can't drive another kilometre. I wake up the next day and hit the road. There's massive relief when I reach Dorrigo to stay with my close friend and organic garden mentor, Jade, and her hubby, Paul, who nurture my shattered nerves and dissipated body, and fill me with the best home-grown organic food and love. I could move in permanently! They're so spoiling me.

A couple more stops, and I arrive back home in Noosa with a car that needs work, but now I need to fly to Sydney to do a course. When I get back, I try to get the car fixed, but it's not possible two days before Christmas. Thankfully, my friends Stephen and Noely swap cars with me, so I can drive safely to Krishna for two weeks. What a swap. I get their new car and give them one that can only travel short distances! This couple is always helping me by fixing my computer, lending me a phone or a car, and sharing a laugh. And I'm staying with them when I return until my next house sit.

My real estate agent shows me a house she says is prefect for me. but I say to her, "I'm so tired, I don't even know if I like it or not."

I spend Christmas at Krishna Village. There are lots of celebrations happening here. On Christmas day, all of the volunteers and guests have a picnic lunch at Mt Warning by the river. It's a fabulous day, so peaceful and multicultural. People from all over the world sing their Christmas songs or share their traditions, and there's a variety of food served.

It's a beautiful, warm day to be on the rocks and in the water. There are no gifts, which makes me happy, as I call Christmas *Unnecessary Consumption.* I feel so 'normal' and relaxed.

For my stay this time, they have me discuss with the chef what's on the menu, and if I can't eat it, he cooks something else for me. I feel so cared for and loved. The beautiful, young, kind cook is always happy to go over the menus with me each morning.

CHAPTER 36

Mold: The Enemy

January, 2018

I'm housesitting in Peregian Springs at a Lyme friend's house. Carole has gone to Cyprus for treatment. It's a welcome relief to have a place to call home for six months. I need to stop and really focus on fast-tracking this wellness thing and get working again. The house is close to the beach, and there are lots of new walking tracks and streets for me to explore. I now have time to slowly build some form of fitness.

I'm dangerously close to a supermarket. It means my sweet tooth has easier access to chocolate and ice-creams, which isn't so good. Yes, I've exposed my weakness! I have an uncontrollable sweet tooth from lunchtime on, especially for chocolate, my go-to when upset … or anytime, really.

The real estate agent takes me to the house again. My head is in a much better space to make decisions, and I'm interested. I go home and do the sums. I could afford this cottage and still support myself for six months. I'm feeling good, so I figure six months is a generous timeframe before I'll be back in the workforce. I check out the house a few more times and purchase it.

A couple of weeks later, I'm diagnosed with mold illness, which explains why I couldn't breathe very well while swimming at the beach the other day, and the surf lifesaver had to rescue me. It was a bit scary to be out there and realise I couldn't swim back. Breathing sometimes feels optional for my body.

My whole world goes into a spin. I fast-track learning about mold. The doctor gets me to order an Environmental Relative Moldiness Index (ERMI) test for my new house, and it comes back high, which means it will continue to make me sick. I hire a building biologist to assess my home, and she gives me a long list of things I need to do before remediation.

I can't believe this is happening. I wish I'd known this before I purchased the house. I'm having a hard time getting my head around this world of mold, which is a whole new complex way of living. The crazy thing is, there isn't anything to see or smell. The house is clean, sunny, and airy. There's no carpet, but it's an old Queenslander, a beautiful wooden house built back in the 1930s, and apparently the combination of a wooden house and the Queensland humidity is a recipe for disaster for mold-affected people. But I love living in the warm climate of South East Queensland, so moving away isn't an option.

I do the remediation, which is a costly exercise involving a company bringing in seven people with industrial air filters/purifiers, fans, and cleaning equipment, to basically sterilize every square millimetre of the house. Thankfully, I haven't moved in yet, and I still have the housesit place. I start getting all of my stuff out of storage. Basically everything has to go, as it will have some (hidden) trace of mold on or in it, but I want to hang onto some precious things, and I need to work out how to do that. I know I should get rid of basically everything, but I'm not working, and money doesn't grow on trees!

I sort my stuff into sterilised by washing machine or dishwasher, donate to charity shop, put into recycling bin, rubbish bin, or sell. I can't bring in anything porous, as it would definitely have mold.

I truly struggle to understand all of this and deal with the grief associated with not being able to bring my special stuff into my home. I must take pictures of the photos and then throw them in the bin, as the photos, as well as all paper and cardboard, are a food source for mold. Plus my furniture, fairly new mattresses, and paintings. The list goes on and on, and all have to go. I can't believe I have to part with so much of my stuff that looks and smells fine, but these are the new rules of my life. Clean, simple, and totally minimalistic. It really does my head in. I think friends and family believe I've really 'lost the plot,' and I do feel a bit that way too as the paranoia sets in. Mold is real and extremely dangerous to your health if you have the mold gene, and it's switched on, which Lyme has done.

I purchase the recommended air purifiers, dehumidifiers, and special heaters, and pay the builder for work he had to do on the house. There goes the money that was meant to support me for six months. I'm back to square one, with no money and only earning a small amount writing for the magazine. This wasn't meant to happen.

There are four things I couldn't part with that were hand-carved especially for me from hardwood. I thoroughly clean them multiple times with special mold cleaner before bringing them into my new home.

My first week in the house, and I'm sleeping on the cold floor on a mat, as I have no furniture. I'm crying and thinking, *What's happening to my fucking life*? Eventually, I order a cheap mattress (not foam), and cheap, colourful furniture. If I can't have quality stuff, I can at least make it look bright and happy.

I argue with the doctor about how new furniture can be better for me with its off-gassing. I often get cross with her in my frustration, because she doesn't seem to understand this added illness and all that it's taking away from me. I just want to get on with my life and have some purpose and meaning.

I feel flat and definitely not excited about my new home, but I need to snap out of it, get stronger and stop fighting with the doctor. I have to remember not to shoot the messenger and that I'm so blessed to have two doctors who know how to treat mold and Lyme. Oh yeah, I now have three doctors at a time. One for Lyme, one for mold, and one is a general GP/MD for day-to-day, non-complicated things ... plus multiple natural therapy practitioners. Appointments are my full-time job. At least with mold, there's a definite treatment pathway/pyramid, but it's expensive. I feel so bad when I get angry at my heart-centred doctor. She's such a lovely lady.

I've been asked to speak at The Diggers Club's Brisbane Tomato Festival in October on both days, as one of the main speakers. Two days is really going push my energy levels, but I'm so excited to be asked, and I accept. It's the perfect focus I need to bring together the speaking course I've been doing in Sydney to create an entertaining, informative talk. Work always provides a positive, meaningful distraction.

CHAPTER 37

The Joining

August, 2018

One of my doctors said, “It’s a great experience having an illness, as we don’t waste our money on mindless things.” *Get fucking real!* Give me back my energy, my work, partying, eating out, having a drink, and travelling overseas, or anywhere, for holidays! I wanted to slap her. How could she make such an outrageous statement when so much has been taken from me, and I’ve lost so many years of my life to illness? Somehow it doesn’t equal an exciting experience like travelling to Africa to sit with gorillas or climbing the Himalayan mountains…things I once did. I do love this doctor. She’s really kind, but she seems a bit out of touch and doesn’t realise how triggering her words are.

Today was my eye specialist appointment, and my little spots are a little bit bigger. I have punctate inner choroidopathy, which basically means that one day a blood vessel in my eye will probably burst, and my vision will be blurry. Then I’ll go into surgery, and they’ll inject something into it, and they repeat it a few more times. It’s a rare eye condition…naturally. Though I’m disappointed with all of the eye supplements I've been taking, I don't focus on this. It's out of my control, and I can't give it any energy. I need to concentrate on getting my body and mind as strong as possible.

I continue going to various appointments and get all of my different treatments, like acupuncture, IR saunas etc., to rebuild my body, and I can feel myself getting stronger. Unfortunately, I'm back to borrowing money from Anne-Maree again, but I've changed my mindset and now say, "I'm grateful my sister wants to invest in my health."

I also must return to government Centrelink payments, but this time I go to the Nambour office, not Noosa, which is helpful and doesn't make me feel bad. I don't know how anyone survives on these payments, even without medical conditions. It would be impossible to get well without any other financial support. I've also decided I need to get back to work, but what exactly would that look like? My body, my energy, my brain, and my days are so unpredictable. I need to earn money again.

I'm getting out and about more, going to horticultural events to keep my knowledge up to date, to Open Gardens, and just enjoying being around people again. I'm also able to retain some more information, though I still get some brain fog, especially with names, and I need to rest often. But I am getting stronger...mentally and physically. I love my new country hometown of Cooran. It's so community-minded, and many people remember me from when I taught the Edible School Gardens program in 2009/10.

I don't have a television to distract me. If I'm not in bed by eight p.m., my body gets cranky and sends a sharp pain shooting through my nervous systems. I then usually can't sleep. So all of this is a fairly good reason to be in bed on time. I read for an hour or two before falling asleep, and the amount of rest I get is unpredictable.

I go to The Joining, a spiritual event about you and your relationships, and attend a group grief session, where there are beautiful, supportive people and lovely ceremonies. When I'm there, I just explode with untapped grief. It pours out of me unexpectedly, and I feel so good for the release, but I'm wiped out for days afterwards.

CHAPTER 38

Tomato Festival

18 October 2018

It's tomato festival weekend in Brisbane. I arrive the day before and stay a five-minute drive from the venue to conserve energy. I have all of my meals and healthy snacks with me and make sure I check everything out, like where I'll be speaking and parking, to make sure I have no stress the next day. It's all about conserving energy, and of course, delivering the best talk.

Before I'm going to speak, I walk away from the crowds, find a quiet space on the grass, ground myself, and just close my eyes for about ten minutes. It does the trick.

I'm the opening speaker, and initially it looks like not many people are coming, but then they pour in. My talk is the best ever. I prepared and practiced heaps, so I'm confident and energised. The information and humour just flow from me. The large marquee is full, and no one leaves. They laugh and join in. I'm so happy with the talk, and people stop me all day and thank me. I'm feeling so good.

The next day, there's a smaller crowd, and the talk doesn't flow as well. Then I'm supposed to do kids' workshops. But it starts to rain, and a huge storm erupts, so I have to stay another night, as I'm wet and totally beat.

It takes a couple of weeks to recover from that, which is a reminder to me that I can't take on too much, and two days of talking plus kids' workshops is way too much. I get excited and say *yes* to events because that's who I want to be again, but it will be my undoing if I don't balance it.

I'm feeling confident about the quality of my talks, though. It's so empowering to be back on stage and get such positive feedback. It makes me strive harder to be disciplined and continue getting stronger in my mind and body.

November 2018

My heart is racing and then missing quite a few beats. The local doctor does an ECG and says they'll monitor it. She thinks it's Lyme-related, but I don't want everything to just be given the Lyme label.

I go back again a month later, again with a racing heart. I'm offered a twenty-four-hour monitor, but I can't deal with the thought of another appointment, because of the amount I've already had this month. I'm tired. I've got so much happening, and my cup is full, so it will have to wait.

I fly to Sydney to do the speaking course that I couldn't finish last time. I've planned everything for minimal stress, but by the time I get there, I'm ready to kill anyone who crosses my path. My heart is beating out of control, and I need food, which is always a problem.

I arrive at the venue late and then go straight out to get a slab of cooked meat (not really a slab, but a lot for me), as I know my body is screaming for protein. I'm like a caveman. I feel better after eating, but my heart is still going crazy.

After the first day of the course, I nearly take myself to hospital emergency, as I'm so worried about my heart, but I don't want to go to a big hospital in a big city, so I put up with it.

Everything else is under control. I have an organic café where I can get food, my accommodation and host are great, and I love the courses. Not only are they educational, but also, I'm away from my strict routines and my Lyme world, and I get to talk to people in a professional way, so I can learn all about their wonderful, exciting dreams and realities.

When I get back home again, I have a quiet Christmas with my daughters, and then it's off to the Woodford Folk Festival, where I'm overseeing kids' workshops with a team of ten people for six days. It's been five years since I last worked here, and I'm anxious. It's really important that we do a good job.

On days four and five, I have to leave the workshops, as I'm absolutely worn out and teary, trying to juggle everything. I must go home and fully rest. I'm frustrated that I can't do what was once so natural for me. I thought I could do it. I pre-prepared all of my meals and don't party at night, but it's too big a challenge to stay in a tent and be woken up as people return from partying at the festival. I return for day six, the last day, but I'm still tired and grumpy. I'm in so much pain by the end, that when I get home, I just fall into bed. It takes me a month to recover.

I loved being back at Woodford Folk Festival, as it's a special place, but it's too much for me. Lots of resting in January does wonders, and my heart starts to calm. My Lyme doctor has prescribed extra magnesium tablets, and that has helped. I'm glad to have no other commitments for a while. *Balance, Leonie. Balance.* My mind is stronger than my body, and that often doesn't serve me.

CHAPTER 39

Dear Diary

Mid 2019

I continue to focus on my primary purpose of regaining my life back, so I listen to health summits all the time on Lyme disease, mold, microbiome, anxiety, and trauma that comes out of the U.S.A. and U.K. They keep me company, inform me of the latest in health and treatments, give my brain some activity, and motivate me.

I've always written a diary, and I encourage everyone who's suffering from a chronic illness to do so, because it's a healing process. When I started writing this book, as I re-read all of my diaries, I cried so much and wondered, on many occasions, how I got through it all. It's a great way to release some of the anger, anguish, despair, distress, fear, frustration, grief, loss, loneliness, pain, sadness, and worry. But it also lets you rejoice in regaining your energy and feeling stronger, healthier, wiser, more joyful, and happy.

It needs to be private, so you can fully express your thoughts. The best thing about diaries is that you can look back and see how far you've come. Acknowledging your progress is so important, because we forget, and what's happening today is the new normal.

You must acknowledge every inch of progress, because each small step forward is a hard-earned win. And you must reward yourself with positivity, happiness, and celebration, no matter how small, and anchor it into your body, mind and soul that you're becoming stronger, healthier, and rebuilding a new you.

I'm excited to notice my brain coming back. I'm remembering horticultural information that I learned and taught years ago. I don't need to write everything down when I listen to a talk now, because I'm confident I'll store that information in my brain and recall it when it's required. This alone has boosted my confidence, especially with work. And though I'll never go back and do my edible school garden programs, as that takes a huge amount of energy I don't have, I'm okay with that now. I was a pioneer in that field, and I'm proud of what I achieved. Today, lots of younger people are running similar programs, and it's their time.

As for me, I'm going to expand into my next passion, which is helping people with chronic illness, especially Lyme disease, get well naturally. I want to make sure they're not alone and forgotten, and get them to realise there are many ways to return your mind, body, brain, and spirit to health, wellness, and positivity.

For years I hid the fact that I was ill, partly because I would cry when I talked about it, but also because I felt like a failure, since I could no longer function in a 'normal' world. It's a tough journey, but I've come out the other side. I'm dreaming again, too. I don't always remember my dreams, but I know I've had them, and that's another positive sign. *Yes... Yes... Yes!* I celebrate each milestone, as I'm winning. We must always celebrate our progress and not focus on the hurdles. Acknowledge them, but move on. Do whatever you have to do to keep moving forward and reaping the benefits of feeling vibrant again.

I'm doing more positive things that will challenge me a bit. I've started going to choir, yoga, and tai chi. I'm constantly expanding my boundaries, slowly, and it's working. I'm also learning to listen to my body. For example, yoga has been too much for me, and I had to find a gentler class. Choir goes to 8:30 p.m. but I can only last until 8:10 p.m., otherwise my body gets really cross with me, and I won't sleep. I won't do tai chi in winter, as I don't like the cold, and I'm slower to get going, I've learned not to rush to get to places anymore. I move slower.

I'm listening to my body and responding. If, for example, I go to someone's home for dinner and get home late, I ensure that in the following few days, I rest fully, with no stress. Working is the same. I'm elated to be back on-stage teaching people about organic gardening and health. It elevates my mental health and sense of wellbeing. But I have to expect there will be consequences and make concessions for it. After I give a talk, I make sure I take extra-special care of myself for the next couple of weeks.

I'm so grateful. I *never* thought I would see the day when I was back on stage doing what I love. Everything is possible. I'm feeling like I'm so close to closing this Lyme chapter of my life.

CHAPTER 40

Same Stuff, Different Day

4 August 2019

Just when I thought I was well and had written the last chapter of this book, I've been infected by another tick! I can't believe this is happening! I realised it when I woke up last night, and my bed was soaked with sweat. There's a lump at the base of my head, which I sort of knew was there, but I was in denial.

I go to a friend's house, and she confirms it's a big fat tick. I phone my doctor straight away--still calm at this moment--and get an urgent appointment with him in the afternoon. The tick drops off before the appointment, but I need to see him for medication.

Two of my doctors sit with me and discuss my options. The first is antibiotics, but they note my body isn't strong enough to deal with them. The other is to increase the amount of Lyme herbs I'm already on, plus some extra ones that Dr Dietrich Klinghardt recommends. I have much respect or Dr Klinghardt, who practises in the U.S.A., Europe, and England, and is a leader in the treatment protocols and latest research of Lyme disease and co-infections.

I can't go through all of this again.

I cry on the way home in disbelief, thinking, *God, stop being so cruel. I don't deserve this!* Once rested and calm, I have an epiphany: I KNOW HOW TO GET WELL! I've been doing it for years.

For the next month, *everything is about me*. I don't allow negative people or energy vampires near me. I have heaps of hyperbaric oxygen therapy (HBOT), colonics, IR saunas, acupuncture, lymphatic massages (my favourite), detox baths, time spent in nature, especially the beach, supplements and potions, and resting. Any time my body starts to get tired, I listen to it, go to bed, and get lots of rest. If I don't, I risk the new Lyme co-infections getting inside my cells, and I sure as hell don't want to go back to being as sick as I was from 2014 onwards. There could be no bigger incentive than knowing the consequences of being slack.

I still question the why and the how of this happening again, and then I laugh! Could it be that the message the Universe was trying to teach me the first time was that I MUST LOVE AND NURTURE MYSELF FIRST? That I needed to protect myself from negative outside influences and be the real Leonie?

This latest tick bite knocked me around for a couple of months, especially with the tiredness, but I got through it by listening to my body and taking care of myself.

CHAPTER 41

Mold Again, Naturally

My doctor wants me to get another Environmental Relative Moldiness Index (ERMI) test on the home I purchased last year and currently live in. I'm not expecting any problems, as everything is in plastic containers. Although, I don't clean as often as I would like, because after doing just one small room, I'm in bed for the rest of the day and definitely am unable to continue on consecutive days.

The ERMI comes back very high. Even higher than before I moved in! I'm shocked. My doctor asks me again if I brought in anything that wasn't new. I had to confess that, yes, I brought in my bedhead, rocking horse, and bookshelves, which are all hardwood. But I explain that I thoroughly cleaned them with high-quality mold cleaners

Then he asks the bombshell question: "Did you clean under the feet of the furniture?" No, I did not. And therein lies the problem. Also, since I've been writing this book, I've had all of my old diaries (and there are lots) spread out all over the floor for weeks/months. The two new mold species prolific in my home are wood and paper. I still can't understand how something so innocent, and particularly my beautiful, handmade hardwood furniture pieces, make my home, and therefore me, sick. I just don't get it. I'm so upset again. How did life get so complicated?

It takes me some weeks to get my head around what this all means to me now. Eventually I come to the conclusion, *I just want to be fully well. Therefore, I will do whatever I have to do, so I can live a life again and be happy, energetic, healthy, and joyful.*

I decide to sell my house. After only sixteen months since moving in. It's such a strenuous time getting my property ready for sale and takes months longer than expected, but I must honour my body when it tells me to stop and rest. As much as I like this cute house, and have a great relationship with my gardening neighbours, I thankfully never got attached to it. I actually made sure I didn't, as I couldn't again endure the grief I experienced when I lost my Cooroibah home, which I still miss.

CHAPTER 42

A Low-Key Christmas

December 2019

I have to fly to Melbourne to visit my daughter, Melika, and my family. I'm so weary before I even leave, between the constant effort of getting the house ready for inspections and hiding most of my health equipment, so people don't think I'm a freak. Having the coffee enema kit in view is probably not a good idea!

I have to take so much with me when I fly. It hasn't become any easier, and I get upset when I start the process on the plane of wrapping the blanket around me and spraying my space. It nearly brings me to tears. I just want to be normal.

I'm in Victoria for only five days, but it's beyond tiring. Being around so many car fumes, noises, chemicals, and eating food I wouldn't normally eat, takes such a massive toll on me, and I must sleep lots. There's too much moving around and too much going on. I take weeks to recover, simply because I'm still so busy when I get home, with Woodford Folk Festival Permakids activities to finalise. I'll be managing and working with a team of nine people for six days, as I did last year.

When I get off the plane at Sunshine Coast Airport, desperate to get to bed, I receive a text from the Permakids team to say they're doing a trial set-up of our bamboo structure for the event, and can I be there in an hour? It's an hour's drive away! I make it, and although I'm desperate for rest, I'm glad to see the magnificent work the team has been doing on our structure. That alone gives me some energy. I'm so relieved to again be home in my little village of Cooran, Queensland.

My daughter Fedora wants to know what's happening for Christmas. I say, "NOTHING! I'm too tired to do anything." This time I really mean it. We settle for toast and avocado smash. I have no energy to be bothered. The bonus is that my daughter, for my Christmas present, cooks all of my meals for me to take to the Woodford Folk Festival. What a blessing. I eat four meals a day. and there isn't a better present for a chronically ill person than precooked food.

CHAPTER 43

Woodford Folk Festival

27 December 2019

Day one at Woodford Folk Festival's kids' permaculture program. It's really popular and a hive of activity. My adrenaline is pumping, and I'm excited. Tonight is the opening ceremony, where tens of thousands of festival people come together to celebrate, but I'm starting to fade.

By the time I get back to my tent at approximately nine p.m., my body is NOT happy. My nervous system is tingling, sending a sharp shooting pain through me, I have heart palpitations, and I'm ready to collapse. Then I lie in bed wondering why I push myself to do these projects.

The next morning, I wake and realise if I'm going to last the remaining five days, I have to drastically change the way I manage myself, or otherwise it will be a repeat of last year, and I'll end up going home early. My solution is that I need to be the team manager only and not get involved with the workshops.

I go to the area in the morning and check that everyone is set up for the day. Then I wait until the workshops begin to make sure all is running smoothly, before going back to my tent, eating a meal, having a short rest, and then returning to catch the workshops in full action. There are joyful, excited, contented children everywhere. And parents, too. I chat with some people and then let the team know when it's time to bring the workshops to a close. I oversee the packing up and enjoy the festival during daylight hours.

Once I eat dinner, I'm in bed for the night. How I would love to be out partying all night, but I accept that I'm lucky to even be here. I've finally learned to prioritise my body's limits and manage to work around that. And believe me, it isn't easy, as I'm so used to doing it all. This is my second year at the festival, and I'm so proud of what I achieve with the Permakids team.

The second of January 2020 is pack-down day at the festival. We must take down the bamboo structure and remove all of our workshop materials from the site. It's always a massive job, and everyone is tired and wants to go home. I must keep sitting, as I don't want to wind up falling down, and it's a hot day. I feel bad, as I probably look like I'm slacking off.

Like I said, to the untrained eye, you would never know I was sick, so people would probably expect me to be pitching in like everyone else and dismantling and packing our cars. My team knows I've got Lyme, and although I shouldn't be doing anything with my body screaming at me to fully rest, I feel guilty. I know we're all tired, and the longer we take to pack up, the hotter it gets. So against logic, I keep getting up and helping. I also need to be here until its finished to make sure everything is done.

It's my birthday. When we stop for morning tea, I find out my good friend Fiona has cooked a birthday cake for me, and the team give me cards and a beautiful spoon necklace. I feel quite emotional. My Permakids team has been so special this year. I'm feeling loved and valued.

CHAPTER 44

Answers

I'm going to a different doctor. I felt I wasn't getting anywhere and needed a new set of eyes with a different focus. Before my first appointment with him, I email a long letter explaining everything he might ever want to know about me, and when I walk in, he's already gone through EVERY blood test I've had since 2014 … and there are lots.

There's much conversation about my gut and an extensive list of blood tests for me to have. Next visit he says to me, "No wonder you're so tired. You have extremely low iron levels. Plus, you're low in a few others like copper and zinc." An intravenous (IV) schedule is booked in. I'll initially get two iron (ferritin), and then magnesium, zinc, and vitamin C every two weeks, until my body picks up.

I'm so relieved to get some answers. I especially need it at the moment, as so much is happening in my life. My house has sold, so I need to sell most of my possessions and then find a van in which to go travelling around Australia. I really don't know anything about vans, but I figure that's my best option while I have the opportunity. I also need to prepare mentally and physically for Fedora's wedding in March.

March 2020

There's a slight spanner in the works. The Covid-19 virus. Oh my goodness. Every day there are new restrictions/rules coming in. Even my doctor's wearing a mask, disposable apron, and gloves. They're closing the clinic for physical visits, so no more IVs. I find it ironic that sick people can't see their doctor. My appointments are to be on Skype, I don't really see the point of that when they're meant to be keeping tabs on my lungs and heart. I also keep getting told I'm a high-risk for Covid.

CHAPTER 45

Time To Celebrate

I'm getting so overwhelmed by everything. My daughter's wedding is in Brisbane in five days, and every day the guest list keeps shrinking as people decide it's too risky. There's no toilet paper in the supermarkets, because people are panic buying (weird), and suddenly we're not allowed to hug our friends or be within 1.5 metres of another human. What's happening to the world?

I'm driving one day and realise I can't cope. I have so much on my plate and must reduce my stress and feelings of being overwhelmed. I decide to quit my much-loved job at Woodford Folk Festival's Permakids. I'd already started planning for the next festival in December, and there's so much work involved. Everyone is shocked.

I quit other things I'm involved with and almost left my job writing for the magazine, but thankfully some logic has prevailed, and I didn't. Writing for the magazine is something I actually enjoy, as it makes me stay proactive with what's happening in horticulture and allows me to keep readers up to date with what to do in their gardens. Plus, when someone asks what I do for work, I can actually give them an answer!

I phone my insightful kinesiologist, Greg, because I can tell I'm heading into meltdown. As usual, he's spot on, quickly identifying how frightened I am. We talk at length about how I can cope with what's going on, and he gives me the usual NCB and PCB statements to work on. It really makes such a positive impact on my mindset. I'm much calmer.

20 March 2020

It's the day before the wedding. I have to take so much with me, including, on this occasion because I'm worried about Covid-19, my two air purifiers to place in the hotel bedroom. It's a two-hour drive to the hotel, and I'm emotional. There's so much happening with this virus thing.

In Brisbane, I meet my daughter, her fiancé, and the bridal party at a pub/café on the river. No one is worried about social distancing. We're all squeezed together around the table. I look around the pub, and no one else is taking any notice, either, which is the complete opposite to what we're being told.

This should have been putting the wind up me with Covid, but I've been craving normalcy, and it's only for a short time, as they all need to head to dinner with other wedding guests for a pre-wedding catch up. I don't go, because I have to conserve my energy. Plus, it's unlikely I'll find food I can eat at the pub, and it will be noisy. I need to minimise exposure to stress.

I don't sleep much, maybe a couple of hours early in the evening, and nothing after midnight. Not a good start to the day.

The makeup artist and hairdresser are in the bride/bridesmaids' hotel room. They're enjoying champagne, and I'm loving watching them and being around the girls.

All is going well. The hairdresser has finished my hair, which is no easy task, because it's thick and long. I ignore how she's spraying so much hairspray, since it's just part of what you do on wedding days, so I ask my body to forgive me. I love the glamour of it all. It's been so many years since I've dressed up for an event, and oh, how I've missed it. I'm excited to finally see my daughter's wedding. Both families are so happy for this loving and well-suited couple. I'm doing well.

By now I'm feeling really tired, and my body would love a sleep, but I can't put my head down on the pillow with my hair just done. Being excited, unfortunately, will exhaust me, too. It's such a delicate balance. My wonderful, loving niece, Mia, arrives to do my makeup back in my room She's always so positive. She chats away until she boosts my energy again. Other healing friends have also been doing some remote reiki and body talk work on me to get me through the day/night. It's a huge day for my body.

I've put on my fabulous dress and high shoes, feeling positive and strong. I want this day to be special for everyone.

Back in my daughters' room, there's a hive of activity as they all get dressed. The photographer is busy capturing the day and then drives me to the church. I think about how this has been the longest wait for a wedding in anyone's life and probably the last one for many months, with all of the restrictions. But right now, none of those matters. I'm feeling tired but excited. My sisters, Anne-Maree and Trish, and my brother, Michael, are here, plus their partners, Peter and Lisa. Mia sits next to me at the wedding and is watching out for me all night, supporting me whenever needed. I'm so grateful to have my family with me.

The wedding is beautiful. Brock and Fedora are such a wonderful couple and will always be together. Brock's parents are family-orientated and happy, and perfect role models.

The night is full of happiness, joy, and fun. My adrenaline kicks in, so I dance heaps and last until 10.20 p.m., which is really late for me, but I'm so glad I've managed the night.

The next morning, I actually wake up feeling great, at least for a couple of hours, before it hits me. It's a long drive home, and I end up stopping on the way for a rest with my friends Merry and Ted, and get a treatment. Though I'm worn out, I'm so happy. The wedding was lovely, and everyone enjoyed the celebration.

CHAPTER 46

A Place To Call Home

I wake two nights later at one a.m. in a panic. My house settlement is in two weeks, and I need somewhere to live ASAP, as no one is allowed to travel anywhere due to Covid.

I get out of bed, because I know I won't be able to sleep now, and start emailing permaculture people I know who have multiple dwellings on their properties. My basic message is, *Help, I need somewhere to stay!* As luck would have it, my friend Colleen will have a cabin free in ten days' time. I didn't even look at it. I'm told it's clean, airy, and the walls are painted with mold inhibiter, so I just write, *Yes, please*, as I know finding accommodation will be difficult, and I have no time to look. Thank goodness for friends.

I have so much to do. All of the people who were going to help me move now can't, because of the Covid restrictions. Plus, I don't want to risk infecting them, as I've been at my daughter's wedding where social distancing was ignored. Also, many of the guests had flown from in from Victoria, and I believe that a lot of germs and viruses circulate in aeroplanes. My body cellular memory is screaming, *Here we go! Packing and on the move again!* But I'm so grateful to have somewhere to move to.

The removalist comes on Good Friday and says to me, "What's your new house like that you're moving to?" I reply, "I haven't seen it!" He gives me a curious look, and I explain I didn't have time to go and check it out.

When I finally get there, I breathe a sigh of relief. My new home is a nine-by-three-metre cabin with decking, surrounded by forest. It's so beautiful, peaceful, and the perfect place for me to fully rest and complete my Lyme and mold journey. I love this place, where there are so many little birds and no noise or traffic, and no neighbours using chemical fragrant laundry detergent or playing loud music. In fact, there are no neighbours at all. Just me and nature. I'm so blessed and grateful to my friends. I hope I can stay for a while.

I also realise I'm not ready to buy a van and travel. I still have some healing to do and need the support of my healers, doctors, IVs, and practitioners. Plus, there's Covid, so anyplace where there would be a crowd of people will be closed. Besides, I want to be settled and have more control/sustainability over my life.

Eventually, I'll find land in Cooran where I used to live, in a quiet space, and build a small hempcrete house, which is the healthiest building material for me to live in. I'm in no hurry, though. I'm so very tired of the constant moving and never feeling like I have a place to call home. I want this next house to be permanent, with extensive organic gardens and animals; I don't want to have to move again, and I've learned from my experience that nothing will go into this new house that has any chance of getting mold on it. I've already discarded most of my possessions, so it won't be difficult. I've learned so much on my massive journey.

CHAPTER 47

Feeling Stronger

April, 2020

I'm in my little cabin. Reception is poor for Internet and phone calls, so I decide instead of getting angry every time I'm home waiting for some wave of Internet to brush by me, I'll turn it into an opportunity to explore the area and start getting some fitness, now that I'm feeling so much stronger.

It's winter, and the weather is perfect for being out and about. I find picturesque scenery to set up my computer and go for a walk around the space, which includes parks, rainforest, and a beach. As soon as I get home, I turn off my computer and phone, so that my expectations for Internet are nil. No expectations equals no stress.

After eight weeks, I finally have a satellite installed on my roof, and I now have Internet access. Oh, how lucky I feel. I love being able to speak with people on the phone at night and listen to health talks during the day. I feel normal again. I'm certainly in no rush to leave this tranquil cabin.

I'm feeling SO STRONG. I have zero stress now. I'm spending a lot of time in nature, sometimes with a friend, but often alone. I like my alone time. My brain is coming back, and I can remember more than I've been able to in years. It's so exciting to feel my brain capacity return. I don't freak out if I go to a supermarket without a shopping list, as I'm likely to remember what I need, especially as that's not where I buy the bulk of my food. It used to be frightening with all its noise, fragrances/chemicals, bright lights, and many aisles and rows of shelves. If I didn't have my shopping list to focus on and follow, I would get totally overwhelmed and have to leave.

My physiotherapist recently said to me, "I remember when you first came to see me years ago. Your body was so fragile, that I was scared I was going to break you when I touched you. And you had no muscle under your skin! Now your body is responding, and I can feel your muscles." This made me feel so good. I knew I was getting stronger, but when someone comments on it, especially when they've been treating me since my early Lyme days, it makes me feel like a hero. It's like, *YES! I AM WINNING!* Compliments always spur me on to do more.

The Doctor's IV clinic has reopened for selected patients, and I'm thankfully one of those. I'm still having IVs every two-to-three weeks to increase my immunity and zinc levels (magnesium, Vitamin C, and zinc). Apparently, all of the stress of the last six months with selling the house, the wedding, Covid-19, moving, and no Internet, has dropped my zinc low. To be honest, I think the IVs have kept me upright.

The other day while I was having my treatment, a lovely girl in her early twenties was also having an IV. Her name is Anita, and she's an intelligent, beautiful woman. I thoroughly enjoyed talking to her. She has Lyme disease as well, and it was obvious she'd done a lot of research. We swapped information about what treatments we do at home and the protocols. I was impressed with how informed she was, as she was new to this current health challenge. Most exciting was her clear purpose regarding her goals, but I could see her achieving them, and I was so excited for her.

I could tell she was really tired, but when she went to leave, they brought the wheelchair in. My heart sank for her. It's so cruel that someone so young is so severely affected by this insidious disease. Being in a wheelchair was always my biggest fear. I'm not afraid of dying but of losing the use of my legs. This amazing young lady will get there, though. She has a purpose, and she's focussed. She will win and be back on her feet again. All it takes is time, money, support, and dedication.

CHAPTER 48

Diving Deep

July, 2020

I really am starting to bounce again, which is a good part of my day, every day. I'm just bursting with happiness. I'm so joyful and positive. When I get out of bed in the morning, I'm singing. My whole body is smiling. It's so good to be alive. Thank goodness I didn't end it. I strongly feel the last part of my complete healing is my emotions.

I know I still have lots of grief and anger around everything this illness has taken from me. I have a new psychologist who finally understands about grief with chronic illness, and a spiritual lady to release what I'm holding in my body, as well as my kinesiologist. I've done family constellations, which was an easy process. What this does is remove all of the people in my family/relationships, past and present, who dump their negative stuff on me. It helps me understand that it's their issues and their problems, and the solution is to let it go. It's powerful stuff. I believe your emotions play a massive part in your ability to get well, and I wish I'd done more of this at the start of my journey.

I don't want all of this negative stuff in my head anymore. It doesn't serve me and never has, but it's not that easy to release. By 'it,' I mean the repeated cycle that keeps me stuck in the same pattern (story).

When you've been in a chronic illness for a long time or experienced trauma, your brain wiring is in a loop. I need to rewire my brain with my new story (goals), new behaviour, and positivity, to create new neural pathways. I've started the Dynamic Neural Retraining System (DNRS) Annie Hopper brain retraining program. It's on DVDs, so it doesn't require any Internet to run, as I'm sensitive to EMF exposure and try to minimise the amount I receive.

It's a six-month program, with a daily hour-long commitment. It doesn't sound like much, but with everything else I have to do to stick with my strict routine, it gets harder as the weeks go on. But I completely understand the repetitiveness is required to reprogram my brain, so the limbic system can get out of its loop and function normally again. Our brains are amazing.

There are two parts of the exercises I really love. One is remembering a happy, positive memory and bringing back every detail of that, and the other is visualising my future that includes a particular event, at a particular time. I have to expand on this for approximately fifteen minutes, and I'm finding it fun, but discipline is required.

My doctor is pleased I've finally got the MRI NeuroQuant done. It's a fascinating process that measures the volume of brain structures to identify in images any neurodegeneration. The images then go to the U.S.A., and a report is back at my doctors a few days later, which gives them a clear assessment of any damage Lyme and mold might be causing. It costs $550 to get it done, but I really value my brain and now understand the true value of it. If your doctor knows about these tests, I wouldn't hesitate to get it done and keep monitoring your brain.

I don't get worried about tests anymore. I fully embrace them as an opportunity to dive deeper into my body and find more solutions to make me healthier and stronger, in order to reduce the number of supplements and potions I take. If a new challenge arises, I just look my doctor in the eyes and say, "We will fix that, won't we?" I know my body is so intelligent, and it wants to heal. I must keep searching for the best solutions.

I have a really big sweet tooth, and I've even been hypnotised by two different practitioners over the years, only to end up eating more. Not helpful. I know it comes down to three things: 1) Making it a habit. My whole life I've had homemade biscuits, cakes and desserts every day. 2) Using it as a reward. 3) Using it for emotional comfort. I tell myself I deserve these treats, as I've been good all day with all of my health food and routines.

I'm still trying to find someone who can snap me out of this habit, as my willpower is zero for this one. It's surprising when I'm so strict on myself all day, and I know sugar of any kind, no matter how 'healthy' it's perceived, isn't good for my body and health. Yet I can't get my head around this one.

I think as I get more energy, and I'm out and about more, I'll be distracted and not interested in a sweet substitute to fill the 'loneliness/feeling sorry for myself' gap. My doctor says it's good for me to eat chocolate… but he doesn't see how much of it I eat.

Besides that, I'm feeling strong. My new gut doctor is getting on top of all of my body's nutritional needs and gut issues. Everything I'm doing inspires me to always take excellent care of my body, as I want, and deserve, a healthy, vibrant life, full of love, joy, happiness, and belonging.

Instead of my usual reaction if someone suggests Lyme is a 'gift,' I've now created a list of the positives that have come into my life because of my complete change of lifestyle. I choose to acknowledge, with much gratitude, the enormous number of healers who have shared their modalities to bring me strength and relief. I'm grateful to know who genuinely loves me with all of their heart and to experience love at such a deep, heart-centred, caring level. I've been given much time to observe nature and watch the clouds, to see a leaf summersault down through the air, to listen to the birds and spend time sitting and becoming friends with them. I get to watch plants grow and notice the fascinating behaviour of insects, and to walk along the beach, watching and listening to the waves. I also get to collect heart-shaped stones and hug a tree or a rock.

I'm so grateful every day that I made it this far. I'm grateful my children are healthy, intelligent, loving, and independent. I'm grateful for music, especially drumming, sound-healing and gongs. I'm grateful for canoeing on the water, while watching the moon rise and the sun set. I'm grateful for hugs, phone calls, flowers, cards, and listening to the rain on the roof. And last but not least, I'm grateful for swimming, walking barefoot, dancing, and especially laughing with friends.

Only when I've done my list do I stop focusing on everything else and realise how wonderful my life really is.

CHAPTER 49

Unleashing My Power

Last year, my best friend Karen, who lives in Melbourne, convinced me to book the Tony Robbins event *Unleash the Power Within.* We were supposed to meet up in Sydney, but because of Covid lockdowns, etc., the event is now virtual. I knew of Tony, but his events never interested me. Well, how misguided I was! This four-day event was life-changing. This man has extraordinary energy and life techniques to take you to a whole new level. I feel like I've released so much negative energy and limiting beliefs and have a brand-new toolbox of coping skills.

Tony has completely rewired my brain to focus on what's important to me, like my service to others and leading by example. He had me dancing so much, and I couldn't believe I wasn't only keeping up, but absolutely enjoying it. I've always loved to dance. The Zoom event went until one a.m., but I had to crawl into bed around 8:30, as I needed my sleep.

Even though I missed a lot, I gained heaps to put my life on track. I feel so extraordinarily positive and am now completely focusing on going forward. My whole body is excited. I can see my future, and I can sense that soon something really big and positive will happen, which would only ever have occurred because of the Lyme journey I've been through. This gives me that 'aha' moment and feeling and makes me grateful for the learning on this long and windy voyage.

I can feel my body getting so strong. I know the true Leonie, without any shackles, has been unveiled. I've discovered who I truly am and who I want to be, and it's awesome! I am a heart-centred, intelligent, caring, difference-maker, who's a truth-seeking, wise woman. I am a naturally vibrant, healthy woman, fully embracing everything I can do in this lifetime, with this incredible body, mind, and soul. I'm stronger, happier, more joyful, and loving than I ever thought I would be…than I ever thought I would experience again in my lifetime. My insight into life is so profound now. I can appreciate how this amazing vessel called a body works, and especially how powerful my heart, mind, body, and brain are.

I look at life and at the world with my eyes wide open, absorbing all of the wonders Mother Nature gifts us and the people to hold our hands and heart along the way. I have an achievable list of FUN prescriptions that consists of things I can be doing now, and each week I'm trying something new to create positive pathways in my brain, with new, happy stories to bring into my life. They're simple actions like walking in nature somewhere I haven't gone before, going on a riverboat, horse riding, and dance lessons...all activities that will stretch me a little but not wipe me out. The most exciting part is that I know I'm going to get even stronger. It's hard to believe how far I've come, so my FUN list expands.

CHAPTER 50

Gratitude

October, 2020

I'm not sure where my life is heading. I'm learning to trust. My goal and purpose are still the same as when I uncurled from the foetal position and took those first physically painful steps from my bed: to learn how to recover from Lyme disease, how to heal naturally, and share this information with others, so they can be vibrantly well again.

I didn't realise at the time just how much time this journey would consume. It certainly has been the biggest project I've ever undertaken, and the toughest, but I've done it, and I'm so goddamn proud of myself. At times I've wanted to give up and end it all, but I didn't. I crawled back out of that black cave and kept fighting, and I've been rewarded.

Every day, from the second I wake up, before opening my eyes, I have so much gratitude and love for my healing sleep and the day ahead … because I never thought I would make it this far. Life looks different. Every day, every hug, every experience, every bird singing, every tree, every dance, every friend…my daughters, my sister, my nieces...everything is a gift I'm extremely joyous and grateful for, and it expands my heart.

My life looks different than it did before Lyme disease. I'll always need a strict diet, supplements, and lots of sleep, and to keep my body clean through lots of detoxing. Also, staying away from toxic relationships and people, drinking clean water, exercising, and lapping up sun and nature. I need to constantly practice self-care and be around people and things that bring me joy while helping me be the best version of myself. But let's face it...if more people did this, there would be a greater amount of health, immunity, love, peace, and happiness in the world. I've come to accept what is and embrace that I've come further than I ever expected. I can still live a fulfilling life helping people and bringing joy, love, and happiness to others and myself.

I'm so proud of what I have achieved.

My life is different, and I'm learning to drop the anger and grief for what has been taken from me, but it isn't easy. My losses are huge and includes my work/business, my home/house, my land, the animals I loved so deeply, my friends, my freedom, an energetic body, money, and time. I can add my daughters to that list, as they really lost their mother for many years. But I've stopped screaming *Why Me* and accept what is. I fully embrace and live each day with joy, happiness, mountains of gratitude and love. And it's all okay. I'm blessed with what I have.

CHAPTER 51

You Can Do It

I need to remind you beautiful Lyme people reading this book that we are some of the most intelligent patients a doctor will ever see, because we have to search out the information for ourselves. Lyme disease isn't acknowledged by the Australian government, or by most doctors or hospitals, so your treatment is already compromised.

You will have to fund your own long recovery from chronic Lyme. You may have to stop working but might not qualify for Centrelink health/sickness benefits, because your illness doesn't exist. It will likely be labelled chronic fatigue, and you will be put onto Jobseeker (formerly Newstart).

You will be rejected from accessing your superannuation if you mention Lyme. You may have to sell your home to pay for extensive and expensive health care or decide which supplements, medication, or treatments you can afford each month.

Overcoming the worst effects of chronic Lyme disease has cost me well over $100,000. Yes, I know how much that hurts. I still miss my home. And so often I think of all the holidays I could have had with that money. However, as another patient said to me, "But you wouldn't have enjoyed it, as you would have been too sick!"

Some friends and family might walk away from you when you need support and love the most, because you can't do what you used to, and they don't understand. This has the ability to shatter your heart and soul if you let it, but don't. Understand that in the long-term, you will be grateful they walked out of your life or stepped back, as it allows new friends who truly love and support you unconditionally to come in.

Life can become lonely, as your capacity to be out in the world is limited, and at first it may feel overwhelming. BUT, I'm here to tell you from experience, you *will* get better, and you will look at life with so much gratitude, because you've learned that the most important thing is your health, and everything else is a bonus.

I hope that writing of my experience has helped thousands of people. There are more support groups starting online. Choose the ones that work for you. Always remember to go with your gut feeling, and if one group doesn't feel right, leave it. If a doctor or health professional's treatment isn't progressing, or you outgrow what they can do for you, find a new one. Listen to health summits online, especially all of the Lyme and mold ones. They will keep you up to date. You are the number one priority.

A quote I love from Anthony Williams (the 'Medical Medium'):

It's not your fault. This isn't karma, and you deserve to be well.
You're so loved and needed by your family,
a friend, and a community,
and we all want you to be the healthiest, most
loving, happiest version of yourself.

He often said this at the end of his podcasts, and I always felt it was for me.

Epilogue

My wish for you is that your journey is much easier. The pathways are already smoothed out for you. Don't be overwhelmed with so much misinformation, that you're sent down the wrong path. I've observed just how attached most people are to their money when they could be rewarded by helping others.

I tried so many treatments in my desperation to get well. You will not have to do this, as you can learn by my trial and errors. They don't all work. Everyone is different, and bodies respond differently. The exciting part is that new technology that's more effective is coming out every year, like bioresonance. Not all treatments cost money. Many are free or cheap processes you can do at home.

My website, *www.LeonieShanahan.com.au*, provides further information on healing processes and how to contact me.

Find your tribe. Find your power. Find your purpose. It's in there, from wanting to grow a fabulous garden, to being a great parent, to being an artist. Become a healer for yourself, or change the world. But most importantly, find the real you.

Your Body Is Designed To Heal. You Deserve To Have A Loving, Healthy, Full Life.

You Are Worthy.

You Are Stronger Than You Think.

Believe In Yourself.

Treatments

These are all treatments I've personally used. Please do not substitute this for medical advice. See your doctor to discuss which ones are right for you.

Asyra bioenergetic machine/treatment

This is used to scan for specific physiologic abnormalities or disease states.

During the Asyra test, patients hold onto two metal probes that are connected to the Asyra machine, which sends specific frequencies throughout the body. These frequencies correlate with particular physiologic abnormalities or disease states.

If the frequencies correspond to specific human frequency signals already present within the body, then that means there's a toxic condition or physiologic abnormality. These conditions often underlie disease states.

Once they're identified, a treatment can be applied to remedy the issue.

Asyra technology does not diagnose or treat any specific diseases but helps to balance and restore normal frequencies of the body, so that it can heal itself naturally.

A Bioresonance machine measures the frequency of energy wavelengths coming from the body. It's based on the idea that unhealthy cells or organs emit altered electromagnetic waves due to DNA damage. The Asyra system gives you an instant response to help you explore the root causes of health problems and how to solve them. This is completed in moments, non-invasively, and with no practitioner bias.

BioMat

A BioMat is a healing 'pad' of amethyst crystals, far Infrared rays (FIR), and negative ions. The mat lies on top of your mattress and converts electricity through a computerised control panel into FIR.

FIR was discovered by NASA to be the safest, most beneficial light waves. They increase blood circulation (where applied) in the human body. Infrared therapy, also known as thermotherapy, results in increased tissue temperature. Thermotherapy also increases blood flow, which makes healing tissue easier on the body by providing nutrients, protein, and oxygen where the healing must occur.

Studies have shown that a one-degree Celsius rise in tissue temperature is associated with a ten to fifteen percent increase in local tissue metabolism. This increase helps healing by eliminating metabolic by-products of tissue damage and supplies an environment for repairing the tissue and supporting a healthy immune system. It decreases your pain and detoxes. The BioMat has seventeen layers, including Amethyst.

More information is available at *www.innerglow.com.au*

Brown's gas

This is water that has been 'enhanced' due to bubbling Brown's gas (BG) through it. A Brown's Gas Generator uses a small amount of electricity to convert the normal liquid water into a complicated gas. Separate sources of hydrogen and oxygen mixed together are called simple gases. Brown's gas is an intricately combined mixture of hydrogen and oxygen.

Coffee enemas

Coffee enemas remove toxins accumulated in the liver and free radicals from the bloodstream. Caffeine travels via the hemorrhoidal vein and the portal system to the liver, opens up the bile ducts, and allows the liver to release bile, which contains toxins. The theobromine, theophylline, and caffeine in coffee dilate blood vessels and bile ducts, relax smooth muscles, and increase the bile flow.

It's best to do your enema next to the toilet with old towels underneath you. The enema bucket should not be more than 45cm (18 inches) above you, to allow a slow flow. While lying on your right side, pull your legs towards your chest in a relaxed position, cover yourself with a blanket to keep warm, and use a pillow to rest comfortably.

The coffee enema is administered to the rectum at body temperature and held for twelve to fifteen minutes, before being released. To begin, you may only want to hold it for five minutes and increase as you get more experienced. If it's difficult to hold the enema, a warm 350mls of distilled water enema can be used first, to empty the colon.

For more information, visit the Gerson Institute website at *https://www.gerson.org*. When you purchase a kit, there will be clear instructions about which coffee to use and how to brew it, as well as the type of water you should use.

It's important to take a binder supplement, for example clay or charcoal, before and after the enema to mop up toxins released from the bile duct. Binders attach to toxins and escort them safely out of the body.

Colonics

Colonic hydrotherapy, or colon irrigation, is the infusion of water and other liquids, such as coffee and minerals, into the rectum. It cleanses and flushes out the colon to remove accumulated waste. You lie on your back and allow the colon therapist to do everything. No mess, no stress, and no cleaning up.

A colonic uses a closed-tube system for taking out the faecal matter, and warm water is released into the colon. The pressure promotes a reflexive contraction of the colon muscles, called peristalsis, which forces waste out of the colon, back through the hose, and into a closed disposal system. There's no smell involved, and you can't see the faecal matter coming out, unless you want to watch it or get a description from your therapist who always love their job and are fascinated by your 'product!'

Deta Elis /Devita Ap

The technology of Bioresonance has evolved into the creation of diagnostic, healing, and prevention devices. Diagnostic equipment can also be used for therapeutic purposes.

The DetaElis AP Bioresonance device has programs with specific frequencies that are used for relieving a stressful burden on the body that can be caused by the presence of parasitic forms such as viruses, bacteria, fungi, protozoa, helminths, and the presence of endo- and exo-toxins, heavy metals, etc., that block the work of the main excretory systems.

When synchronised exactly, these frequencies, or vibrations, cause the micro-organisms to absorb this energy and make them vibrate until their outer shell or wall is broken, and they're no longer active.

The device includes a range of basic complexes consisting of manual and automatic programs. Each user can create their own unique complexes (the whole device can hold up to fifty) and has the ability to download new complexes and programs that are created by the company's specialists. The small device hangs around your neck.

You can find out more details at *https://detaelis-bioresonance.com*

Dry brushing

Dry body brushing works by exfoliating the skin. You rub a brush with coarse, natural-fibre bristles over your body in a particular pattern towards your heart.

This may help boost the lymphatic system by stimulating and encouraging blood flow and circulation

Hyperbaric oxygen therapy (HBOT)

This involves the breathing in of oxygen at a greater-than-normal pressure. It increases the level of oxygen at a cellular level and oxygenates the blood, leading to faster healing and reduced inflammation, thus increasing the amount of available oxygen to the tissues and then restoring them. HBOT looks like a space shuttle that you lie inside.

Hyperthermic Ozone and Carbonic Acid Transdermal Therapy (Hocatt™)

This hyperthermia treatment with ozone may promote immunity, energy, and detoxing. No medical practitioner should ever take their patient over forty-two degrees.

Light therapy (Wellbeam)

This involves Near-Infrared therapy at 850nm and 660nm Red.

It's beneficial for wounds, injuries, pain relief, respiratory difficulties, and immunity.

Ionic footbath

This removes heavy metals from your body, which is a priority for healing to progress.

The ionizing machine works to ionize the foot bath water, and pull toxins out of your body through your feet. This process is said to give the hydrogen in the water a positive charge, creating a liver detox and purge heavy metals. Benefits include a liver, kidney, and parasite cleanse, which enhances your immune system and improves your memory and sleep.

You can find out more details at *https://kiscience.com*.

Lymphatic exercise mini trampoline

The lymphatic system does not have a pump in the body, and therefore you need to keep it moving by exercising.

You can find out more information at *www.innerglow.com.au*

Lymphatic massage/lymphatic drainage

This is a gentle, rhythmic massage treatment performed by a specialist trained in lymphatic massage, which stimulates the circulation of lymph fluid around the body. The physical stimulation helps rapidly speed up the removal of wastes and toxins from a sluggish lymphatic system. It may even provide a significant boost to your immune system.

Lymphatic massage aims to increase the efficiency of your lymphatic and circulatory system and enhance your circulatory system's capacity to rapidly remove retained fluids and any toxic waste build-ups, improve circulation, increase metabolic rate, and has the potential to enhance your immunity.

Lymphatic neck massage

Dr Klinghardt's lymphatic neck and throat massage for drainage and brain detoxification.

You can find out more information at *https://www.sophianutrition.com/blogs/sofia-life-blog/lymphatic-throat-massage.*

MRI NeuroQuant

This is for patients presenting with symptoms relating to memory and cognition. It provides an objective measure of brain volume, specifically of brain structures commonly damaged by Alzheimer's disease.

It then compares these volumes to a national database of patients of the same age, sex and skull size who have healthy brains. With this information, NeuroQuant provides you and your healthcare team with a valuable tool in the workup for patients who have mild, moderate, or severe cognitive impairment.

NeuroQuant can increase your confidence that the symptoms are due to neuronal loss rather than other possibilities, including medication side effects, anxiety/depression, sleep apnoea, or nutritional deficiency, among others.

Neti pot

The Neti pot is a fluid-filled vessel that looks like a teapot. It's used to flush or rinse the sinuses and nasal passages with warm water.

A sinus flush, also called nasal irrigation, is usually done with saline, which is just a fancy term for salt water. When rinsed through your nasal passages, the saline can wash away allergens, mucus, and other debris, and help to moisten the mucous membranes.

Ozone

Ozone treatments are highly valued for various effects. You buy the ozone machine and oxygen, and do it yourself at home. It's important to follow the instructions (all online) correctly. Ozone insufflation can even be used in the vagina and rectum.

The benefits include being antimicrobial, increased oxygen in your body, pain relief, immunity modulation, improved antioxidant levels, increased ATP production, anti-inflammatory properties, and improved elasticity of red blood cells.

The benefits of ozone therapy clearly state its usefulness in treating a myriad of pathologies, as well as enhancing general well-being.

You can find out more information *at http://o3academy.com.*

10-Pass Ozone

This method is when 200–220ml of a patient's blood is drawn under negative pressure (vacuum). The blood is then mixed under positive pressure with 200ml of ozone at a concentration of 70 ug/ml, and then re-infused into the patient's vein, also under positive pressure.

Pulsed Electro Magnetic Field Therapy (PEMF)

This is an alternating electrical current used to produce an electromagnetic field. It may induce healing and works to reduce pain, inflammation, the effects of stress on the body, and platelet adhesion. It also improves energy, circulation, blood and tissue oxygenation, sleep quality, blood pressure and cholesterol levels, the uptake of nutrients, cellular detoxification, and the ability to regenerate cells.

PowerTube®

This device works on the skin and cycles through three stages that use high frequencies. It rebalances the body by creating wellness and homogenisation of the molecular structure of blood, which strongly enhances your ability to heal and provides relief. Alternating current and frequencies correspond to the water molecule.

Reiki

A Japanese technique for stress reduction and relaxation that also promotes healing. It's administered by 'laying on hands' and is based on the idea that an unseen 'life force energy' flows through us and is what causes us to be alive.

SCIO biofeedback machine

The machine scans your body like a virus-scan on a computer, looking for anything from viruses, deficiencies, weaknesses, allergies, abnormalities, and food sensitivities. It gives you information about your body on an energetic level, reports on the biological reactivity and resonance in your body, and indicates needs, dysfunctions, and vulnerabilities.

Suggested Routines

It has taken me more than six years to come up with these routines. I didn't know any of it when I first started. I mainly slept the first couple of years.

Obviously, I don't always achieve all of this in a week. and that's okay. You can only do so much.

These suggestions are based on what I've discovered has worked for me. It isn't medical advice. Please do your own research to figure out what methods work best for you and your lifestyle.

Breathing

Remember to breathe long, slow, deep breaths down into your belly several times during the day.

Upon waking

I like to wake up with the birds, so I can enjoy their birdsong. It makes my heart sing.

While still in bed:

- Check in with yourself to figure out if you had any dreams and if you did, were there any messages in them? (For many years after getting Lyme, I didn't dream.)

- Think of six things to be grateful for. Examples include your bed, sleep, birds singing, the peaceful country, your legs that hold you up, your arms that hold your cup, clean water, friends.
- Visualise your day and how you want it to play out.
- Check in with your body. How is it feeling? Do you need to rest more? Do you have some energy?

On rising and before breakfast

- Use a tongue scraper or a teaspoon to scrape the toxins and bacteria off the top and sides of your tongue and then rinse. Once you start this practice, your mouth will feel so good, you won't want to live without it.
- Splash your face with cold water. In the summer, I keep water in the fridge for this.
- Go outside, and look at the sun. Then close your eyes and take a few slow breaths.

Open your eyes again, and, stand barefoot on the ground (this is called earthing), and take deep breaths. Blow all of the old air out of your body, and expand your lungs.

- Put your hands on your sternum (chest), and do gorilla pumps to stimulate the thymus gland and increase your life force energy. (Also do this before bed).
- Do some yoga, especially cat stretches (outside, when possible).
- Jump on a lymphasiser trampoline.
- Do oil pulling for twenty minutes.

Start with 1 teaspoon of warm coconut oil before increasing to one tablespoon as you get used to the flavour and texture.

Put the oil in your mouth, and swirl it around for ten to twenty minutes. Then spit it into an old container to dispose of in the rubbish when full. Do not spit into the basin or sink, or it will clog your drains.

Oil pulling draws toxins out of your mouth and improves the health of your gums and teeth.

- Do a Neti pot nasal rinse (4-5 times a week). It's a strange thing when you first start pouring liquid through your nostrils like some party trick, but stick with it, as it totally clears your sinuses. Breathe easy!!

Daily

Walk for at least twenty minutes every morning. Go early, before the sun gets hot, so you don't need sunscreen. Get sunshine on as much of your body as possible to boost your Vitamin D levels.

Before showering, apply a body brush on your dry skin. Only use soap on smelly or dirty bits, as it interferes with Vitamin D absorbing into your skin. Also put a filter on your shower if you wash with town water, as your skin absorbs the chemicals, and you inhale them through the steam in hot showers or baths.

After cleaning your teeth, gargle some water to activate the vagus nerve. Humming and singing will also do this. I sing lots these days.

Use a 'squat stool.' It sits against your toilet, so your knees are raised higher than your hips. This is a natural position for your bowels to expel.

Drink clean water all day to stay super hydrated. Whether you have town water (chemically treated) or rainwater (anything could be living in there), you need to have a filter, and it must be changed regularly, otherwise it becomes unhygienic. There are lots of different filters at varying prices. Do your research to find the best one for you.

Eat organic or biodynamic food. Non-organic food may have traces of glysophate, which is so damaging and harmful to your body.

Store food in glass containers, and drink from glass or stainless-steel containers. Avoid plastics.

Drink tea. I recommend

- Cistus Incanus
- Lemon myrtle
- Lemongrass
- Liquorice root
- Taheebo/Pau d'Arco.

Detoxing

Do as much as achievable each week to keep your body as clean as possible and take the pressure off your organs. Home treatments include:

- castor oil packs
- coffee enemas
- detox bath
- ionic foot bath
- lymphasiser trampoline
- IR sauna
- ozone insufflation. *(Please refer to of the Treatments section).*

Practise meditation and mindfulness during the day, and do lots of slow breathing. Breathe in for a count of four, hold for six, out for eight.

During the day, run air filters, air dehumidifiers, and an oil diffuser.

Get EMF protection for your home, and also one to carry with you. Turn off your router whenever possible. Prevention is better than the cure. Never take your electronic devices, such as your phone, tablet, or computer, into the bedroom at night. Your bedroom is meant to be a hygienic, rejuvenating place for your brain and body to rebuild.

Before bed/bedtime

Watch some comedy. Laughter is so important for your health.

Use your journals. If you've had a bad day, get out your 'negative' journal, and write down everything that pissed you off. Then ask the universe to fix it while you sleep. This journal does not live in your bedroom, which is for sleep and harmony.

Write in your gratitude diary. You can always find lots to be grateful for.

Sleep when you're tired. You probably know your body's threshold at this point.

If you have one, sleep on a Biomat.

If you're having trouble falling asleep, visualise in as much detail as possible about your future healthy self, the wonderful things in your life, the places you'll be going, and what you'll be doing (all positive). Everything is possible in your imagination.

Play calming music.

Positive actions

Before eating, say a grateful prayer over the healthy food that's making your body stronger and healthier.

When taking supplements and potions, once again, give gratitude. Place your hands above them, and thank Mother Earth, the wise elders, scientists, and healers for bringing you these supplements to take your body to the next level of health. Ask the supplements to be of the highest potency for you.

Then put your hands on your body, and ask it to accept these supplements and potions and take them where they're required for maximum absorbency and to make you even stronger. Then pump your sternum and the air in victory!

If you only have a couple of supplements to take and know what each one is going to help you with, give gratitude to each tablet/potion separately, thanking them for their purpose.

Gratitude and love are the highest vibration, and if you can bring more vibration or energy into your supplements/food/body just by giving thanks, then why not do it?

Thoughts change the chemical makeup of your body. Be positive, be grateful, and raise your love vibration.

Use essential oils. Good-quality ones. There are a lot of incredible oils that offer so much for your health. Here are some of my favourites.

- At night, put lavender on the tops of your big toes (relates to your brain), on your wrists, and behind your ears for relaxation.
- Put oregano on your feet, spine, and back of the neck for parasites and mold, and frankincense under your tongue and

nose, as well as across your forehead, for sleep and immunity. Use peppermint for headaches, nausea, fever, and pain, and rosemary for brain and memory.

Make a brew in a jar with sesame seed oil, and add a few different essential oils to spread all over your body during the day.

Positive messages

Write affirmations, and leave them around the house. You might even try angel/tarot cards. Subscribe to Esther Hicks' emails, or get messages sent to your phone.

The non-negotiables!

- Do not consume grains, dairy, alcohol, town water, soft drinks/soda, sugar, big fish and farmed fish, GM foods, junk food, processed foods, and vegetable oils.
- No smoking.
- Never bring chemicals into your house. This includes cleaning products, laundry detergent, perfume, etc. Use only natural products on your body, in your mouth, and in the bathroom, bedroom, kitchen, and laundry.
- Open the doors and windows, and have fresh air moving through your home.

In summary

Yes, there's a lot on this list. But if you want to live a full life again, it takes work. Push your body and mind a little bit more to see what you can get away with. If you don't, you won't know your true capabilities. I'm living proof that you can keep moving forward and win.

Listen to your body, and do what you can, slowly adding more into your routine. Remember that it's designed to heal.

You must feed your body, mind, soul, and spirit to rebuild the new you.

Doctors And Health Practitioners I Highly Recommend

Dr Jay Davidson (Lyme summits)	*https://drjaydavidson.com*
Dr Dietrich Klinghardt	https://klinghardtinstitute.com
Dr Christine Schaffner	*www.sophiahi.com*
Dr Neil Nathan	*https://neilnathanmd.com*
Dr Richard Schoeffel OAM, MD	*https://fullertonhealthmedicalcentres.com.au*
Dr Richard L. Horowitz	*https://lymeconnection.org*
Evan Brand	*https://www.evanbrand.com*
Dr Nicole McFadzean/Ducharme	*https://restormedicine.com/naturopathic-care*
Dr Raj Patel	*http://drrajpatelonline.com*
Dr Darin Ingels	*https://dariningelsnd.com*
Scott Forsgren	*https://www.betterhealthguy.com/lyme/my-story*
Dr Kenneth Stoller	*www.hbotsr.com/services/lyme*
Todd Watts	*https://microbeformulas.com/pages/dr-todd-watts*

Bryan Rosner	*http://www.lymedisease.org/bryan-rosner-supercharge*
Connie Strasheim	*https://conniestrasheim.org*
Greg Lee	*https://goodbyelyme.com/about-greg-lee*
Dr Datis Kharrazian	*https://drknews.com*
Stephanie Seneff (glysophate)	*https://stephanieseneff.net*
Jeffrey Smith (GMOs)	*www.responsibletechnology.org* *Lyme Associations*
Lyme Association of Australia	*https://www.lymedisease.org.au*
Lyme Association of USA	*https://lymediseaseassociation.org*
The International Lyme and Associated Diseases Society (ILADS)	*https://www.ilads.org*
The National Capital Lyme Disease Association	*https://NatCapLyme.org*

Mold

Dr Margaret Christensen (Mold summit)	*https://carpathiacollaborative.com/dr-margaret-christensen/*
Cheryl Ciecko	*https://www.avoidingmold.com/about-me*
Dr Jill Carnahan	*www.jillcarnahan.com*
Dr Jill Crista	*https://drcrista.com*

Mold

Dr Ritchie Shoemaker	*https://www.survivingmold.com*
Dr Sandeep Gupta	*https://www.moldillnessmadesimple.com/about-drgupta*

Various topics

Dr Keesha Ewers (trauma)	*www.drkeesha.com*
Kiran Krishan (mitochondria)	*https://microbiomelabs.com/home/education*
Trudy Scott (Anxiety)	*http://www.antianxietyfoodsolution.com*
Niki Gratrix	*https://nikigratrix.com*
Alex Howard	*https://www.alexhoward.tv*
Dr Nasha Winters	*https://www.drnasha.com*
Donna Gates	*https://bodyecology.com/articles*
Sayer Ji	*https://www.greenmedinfo.com*
Bruce Lipton (the biology of belief)	*https://www.brucelipton.com*
Dr David Jockers	*https://drjockers.com*
David Perlmutter (brain)	*https://www.drperlmutter.com*
Dr Norman Dodge (brain)	*www.normandoidge.com*
Dr Dale Bredesen	*https://www.apollohealthco.com/dr-bredesen*
Dr Anne Louise Gittleman	*https://annlouise.com*

Various topics

Dr Joseph Mercola	*https://www.mercola.com*
Dr Mark Hyman	*https://drhyman.com*
Dr Amy Myers	*https://www.amymyersmd.com*
Nick Polizzi	*https://www.thesacredscience.com/author/nicpol3*
Ty & Charlene Bollinger	*https://thetruthaboutcancer.com/*
Lloyd Burrel (EMF 5G)	*https://www.electricsense.com*
James & Laurentine Food Matters	*https://www.foodmatters.com*
Nick Orton (tapping EFT)	*http://www.nickortner.com/*
Mike Adams	*https://www.healthranger.com/index.asp*

Oral health

Jonathan Landsman	*https://www.naturalhealth365.com/*
Nadine Artemis (her book)	*www.bookdepository.com/Holistic-Dental-Care-Nadine-Artemis*
Dr David Minkoff	*https://www.drminkoff.com/*
Dr Bruce Fife	*http://www.coconutresearchcenter.org*
Dr Thomas E. Levy	*https://www.peakenergy.com/*

Other Books From Leonie Shanahan

Eat your Garden: Organic Gardening for Home and Schools

Elevate Your Energy: The Most Inspiring Way to Take Your Energy to the Next Level

Also available at www.LeonieShanahan.com.au:

Edible School Gardens DVD, an educational step-by-step process for organic gardening.

www.ingramcontent.com/pod-product-compliance
Lightning Source LLC
Chambersburg PA
CBHW062132020426
42335CB00013B/1185

* 9 7 8 1 9 2 5 4 7 1 5 4 0 *